WITHDRAWN

Developing Effective Physical Activity Programs

Physical Activity Intervention Series

Lynda Ransdell, PhD, FACSM

Boise State University

Mary K. Dinger, PhD, CHES, FACSM

University of Oklahoma

Jennifer Huberty, PhD

University of Nebraska at Omaha

Kim Miller, PhD, CHES

University of Kentucky

LIVERPOOL
JOHN MOORES UNIVERSITY
AVRIL ROBARTS LRC
TITHEBARN STREET
LIVERPOOL L2 2ER
TEL. 0151 231 4022

LIVERPOOL JMU LIBRARY

an Kinetics

3 1111 01297 8399

Library of Congress Cataloging-in-Publication Data

Developing effective physical activity programs / Lynda Ransdell ... [et al.].
    p. cm. -- (Physical activity intervention series)
  Includes bibliographical references and index.
  ISBN-13: 978-0-7360-6693-8 (soft cover)
  ISBN-10: 0-7360-6693-4 (soft cover)
  1. Physical fitness. 2. Exercise. I. Ransdell, Lynda.
  GV481.D46 2009
  613.7--dc22

                    2008045911

ISBN-10: 0-7360-6693-4 (print)   ISBN-10: 0-7360-8541-6 (Adobe PDF)
ISBN-13: 978-0-7360-6693-8 (print)   ISBN-13: 978-0-7360-8541-0 (Adobe PDF)

Copyright © 2009 by Lynda Ransdell, Mary K. Dinger, Jennifer Huberty, and Kim Miller

All rights reserved. Except for use in a review, the reproduction or utilization of this work in any form or by any electronic, mechanical, or other means, now known or hereafter invented, including xerography, photocopying, and recording, and in any information storage and retrieval system, is forbidden without the written permission of the publisher.

Notice: Permission to reproduce the following material is granted to instructors and agencies who have purchased *Developing Effective Physical Activity Programs:* pp. 42, 55, 73, 116, 162. The reproduction of other parts of this book is expressly forbidden by the above copyright notice. Persons or agencies who have not purchased *Developing Effective Physical Activity Programs* may not reproduce any material.

The Web addresses cited in this text were current as of October 16, 2008, unless otherwise noted.

Acquisitions Editor: Michael S. Bahrke, PhD; **Developmental Editor:** Kathleen Bernard; **Assistant Editor:** Jillian Evans and Nicole Gleeson; **Copyeditor:** Patsy Fortney; **Proofreader:** Kathy Bennett; **Indexer:** Joan K. Griffitts; **Permission Manager:** Dalene Reeder; **Graphic Designers:** Bob Reuther and Joe Buck; **Graphic Artist:** Denise Lowry; **Cover Designer:** Keith Blomberg; **Photographer (cover):** © image100/Corbis; **Photographer (interior):** © Human Kinetics, Inc., unless otherwise noted. Photo on p. 3: Bill Crump/Brand X Pictures; photo on p. 23 courtesy of Tim Fitzgerald; photo on p. 35: Bananastock; photo on pp. 60 and 145: George Doyle/Stockbyte/Getty Images; photo on p. 71: Getty Images/Brand X; photo on p. 83: Amy Eckart/Taxi/Getty Images; photo on p. 107: TAUSEEF MUSTAFA/AFP/Getty Images; photo on p. 123: Purestock/Getty Images; **Photo Asset Manager:** Laura Fitch; **Photo Office Assistant:** Jason Allen; **Art Manager:** Kelly Hendren; **Associate Art Manager:** Alan L. Wilborn; **Illustrator:** Alan L. Wilborn; **Printer:** United Graphics

Printed in the United States of America   10 9 8 7 6 5 4 3 2 1

Human Kinetics
Web site: www.HumanKinetics.com

United States: Human Kinetics, P.O. Box 5076, Champaign, IL 61825-5076
800-747-4457
e-mail: humank@hkusa.com

Canada: Human Kinetics, 475 Devonshire Road Unit 100, Windsor, ON N8Y 2L5
800-465-7301 (in Canada only)
e-mail: info@hkcanada.com

Europe: Human Kinetics, 107 Bradford Road, Stanningley, Leeds LS28 6AT, United Kingdom
+44 (0) 113 255 5665
e-mail: hk@hkeurope.com

Australia: Human Kinetics, 57A Price Avenue, Lower Mitcham, South Australia 5062
08 8372 0999
e-mail: info@hkaustralia.com

New Zealand: Human Kinetics, Division of Sports Distributors NZ Ltd., P.O. Box 300 226 Albany North Shore City, Auckland
0064 9 448 1207
e-mail: info@humankinetics.co.nz

CONTENTS

PART I Thinking About the Foundations of Physical Activity   1

CHAPTER 1 Promoting and Maintaining Health Through Physical Activity Recommendations 3

CHAPTER 2 Planning and Evaluating Physical Activity Programs 13

CHAPTER 3 Measuring Physical Activity 23

SERIES PREFACE

The purpose of the Physical Activity Intervention Series is to publish texts, written by the leading researchers in the field, that provide specific and evidence-based methods and techniques for physical activity interventions. These books include practical suggestions, examples, forms, questionnaires, and intervention techniques that can be applied in field settings.

Many health professionals who currently provide exercise advice and offer exercise programs use the traditional and structured frequency, intensity, and time (FIT) approach to exercise prescription. Although the exercise prescription is valid, going to a fitness facility and participating in such programs are not attractive to many people. Alternative programs based on the new consensus recommendations and using behavioral intervention methods and techniques are needed.

The books in the Physical Activity Intervention Series provide information, methods, techniques, and support to the many health professionals—clinical exercise physiologists, nutritionists, physicians, fitness center exercise leaders, public health workers, and health promotion experts—who are looking for alternative ways to promote physical activity that do not require a rigid application of the FIT approach. It is to meet this need that Human Kinetics developed this Physical Activity Intervention Series.

The series has a broad scope. It includes books focused on after-school programs for children and youth, ways to implement physical activity interventions in the public health setting, and ways to evaluate physical activity interventions. The series also includes books that focus on the implementation of interventions based on theories and on interventions for other special populations such as older adults and those with chronic disease. Each book is valuable and useful in its own right, but the series will provide an integrated collection of materials that can be used to plan, develop, implement, and evaluate physical activity interventions in a wide variety of settings for diverse populations.

PREFACE

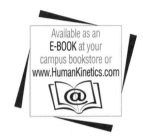

Available as an E-BOOK at your campus bookstore or www.HumanKinetics.com

Anyone interested in increasing physical activity and improving health and fitness should understand several basic terms that will be used throughout this book. *Physical activity* is any bodily movement that results in increased energy expenditure (Caspersen, Powell, & Christenson, 1985). Examples of physical activities include biking or walking to work, taking the stairs instead of the elevator, dancing, and gardening. *Exercise* is planned, structured activity that is designed to improve physical fitness (e.g., cardiorespiratory fitness, muscular strength and endurance, flexibility, and body composition). Examples of exercise include jogging, lifting weights, and swimming laps.

Physical activity and exercise differ in both intensity and desired outcome. The intensity for physical activity can be moderate to vigorous, whereas the intensity for exercise is typically vigorous. The desired outcomes for physical activity and exercise may be slightly different. The desired outcome for physical activity is to improve health and increase resistance to hypokinetic disease, whereas the goal of exercise is typically to improve physical fitness and often athletic performance.

That being said, it is also important to note that at the turn of the century, the U.S. government published *Healthy People 2010* with the intention of setting goals and objectives for improving the nation's health in a variety of areas including physical activity and fitness (*Healthy People 2010 Midcourse Review,* 2005). To date, none of these goals have been reached, although American adults have moved closer to some of their targets (*Healthy People 2010 Midcourse Review,* 2005).

One of the reasons physical activity has not increased substantially in the U.S. population is that physical activity interventions have used a one-size-fits-all approach. However, it is reasonable to assume that women have different activity preferences than men, older adults have different activity preferences than younger adults, and certain ethnic minority groups have activity preferences that are different from those of the dominant culture. For example, compared to men, women tend to prefer group activities such as aerobic dance and lower-intensity activities such as walking, whereas men prefer team sports and higher-intensity activities (Ransdell, Vener, & Sell, 2004). When compared to their younger counterparts, older adults prefer lower-intensity activities that provide a social outlet and offset the process of aging (Allender,

2006). Native Americans tend to participate in culturally relevant activities (e.g., sheep shearing, gardening, traditional dance) in contrast to their white counterparts, who love their yoga classes, sports, and conditioning activities (Ainsworth, Irwin, Addy, Whitt, & Stolarczyk, 1999).

Given the public health challenge to find ways to increase physical activity and to recognize that all populations do not respond to the same type of physical activity intervention, the purpose of this book is to provide evidence-based recommendations for designing more effective physical activity interventions in a number of populations. In *Healthy People 2010 Midcourse Review* (2005), the authors conclude that: "The lack of evidence-based practices for physical activity programs targeting select populations continues to challenge public health practitioners trying to affect physical activity behaviors." Our main objective with *Developing Effective Physical Activity Programs*, is to simplify the process of using evidence-based practices by making specific recommendations for designing, implementing, and evaluating physical activity interventions.

Developing Effective Physical Activity Programs is designed for state health department employees, community program designers, fitness club professionals, and academic professionals. Specifically, anyone interested in training people to design, implement, and evaluate physical activity interventions or conduct research related to physical activity interventions will find this publication valuable.

The introduction of the book provides background information such as common principles for designing any intervention. Part I of the book, Thinking About the Foundations of Physical Activity, then builds on that introductory material by addressing physical activity recommendations (chapter 1), planning and evaluating physical activity programs (chapter 2), and effectively measuring physical activity (chapter 3). Part II of the book, Working With Specific Populations, presents evidence-based recommendations for working with women (chapter 4), obese or overweight people (chapter 5), older adults (chapter 6), and ethnically diverse populations (chapter 7). Part III, Considering the Variables, covers environmental approaches to increasing physical activity (chapter 8), how setting (e.g., home and family, church, medical community, or worksite) can influence an intervention (chapter 9), and using mediated programming to extend the reach of an intervention (chapter 10).

Until now, no single book has covered so many special populations and considerations that can affect the success of a physical activity program. This book stands out because it addresses the unique needs of people who are most likely to be sedentary and who would benefit from a physical activity program. This book recommends evidence-based practices that can significantly improve physical activity interventions in a variety of populations, and it encourages the practitioner to move beyond the one-size-fits-all mentality.

To effectively use this book, a planner should first consider the population for whom the intervention is designed. For example, someone designing a program for African American women should first read the introduction, which outlines several basic principles for increasing physical activity in any population. After reading the introduction, the planner should find chapter 4 (Interventions for Women) and chapter 7 (Interventions for Ethnically Diverse Populations) helpful. If a planner also wants to consider making this a mediated program, chapter 10 provides valuable information. The planner can pick and choose which chapters to read, depending on the population for whom the intervention is designed. The idea is to combine and synthesize information from a variety of chapters to customize a program so that it is likely to succeed.

INTRODUCTION

Collective wisdom dictates that a specific "road map," or plan, should be developed prior to implementing a physical activity intervention. We recommend beginning the program planning process with the following general steps, regardless of the population, setting, or other unique characteristic of the intervention: (a) establish a theoretical basis, (b) use effect sizes from meta-analyses, and (c) use focus groups.

Establish a Theoretical Basis

One of the most important factors in designing a successful physical activity intervention is grounding it in theory. Even today, many interventions are conducted without a theoretical basis or with minimal inclusion of theory. According to Kerlinger (1986, as cited in Glanz, Rimer, and Lewis, 2002) (p. 25), a theory is a "set of related concepts that present a systematic view of events by specifying relations among variables in order to explain and predict events or situations." Theories are generalizable to a variety of people and testable via reasonable means. They specify relationships among variables and guide the search for modifiable factors related to behavior change. A model is a combination of theories and is designed to be more complex and explanatory than a theory.

In this book, using theory means using information from an existing health behavior change theory or model (e.g., the social cognitive theory, transtheoretical model, health belief model, or ecological model). One example of using theory to guide an intervention is the use of social cognitive theory to guide the DAMET study (Ransdell, Oakland, & Taylor, 2003). In the DAMET study (Ransdell et al., 2003), the 11 constructs of social cognitive theory were addressed through specific activities in the intervention. For example, to address the construct of *environment,* girls and women in this study participated in activity in a female-only environment that encouraged group interaction and mixed age and ethnic groups. The construct of *self-control* was addressed by asking mothers and daughters to complete behavioral contracts and physical activity logs, set goals, and role play the process of overcoming barriers to participation in activity.

Cox (2003); Pinto and colleagues (2002); and Bock, Marcus, Pinto, and Forsyth (2001) used the transtheoretical model to plan and implement their interventions. Participants' stage of change (e.g., precontemplation, contemplation, preparation, action, maintenance, termination) was ascertained using a questionnaire. Once the stage of change was established, specific processes of change were used to facilitate increases in physical activity. For example, those in the contemplation stage were encouraged to use experiential processes such as self-reevaluation (i.e., perceiving oneself with and without sedentary behavior). Those in the action stage were encouraged to use behavioral processes such as developing helping relationships (i.e., a buddy system or counselor calls) and practicing stimulus control (i.e., removing cues to unhealthy behavior and adding cues for healthy behavior).

Decisional balance, or examining the benefits of versus the barriers to increasing physical activity, was also examined. As the perceived benefits of exercise increased and barriers decreased, the likelihood that a person would exercise or participate in physical activity more regularly increased. Self-efficacy, or situation-specific self-confidence, was measured via questionnaire as well. A variety of intervention activities were designed to increase self-efficacy. As self-efficacy improved, the likelihood of increasing or maintaining physical activity was enhanced.

Using theory can also mean combining information from data-based studies or various theories or models (or both) to design the most effective program possible. For example, data (i.e., effect sizes) from meta-analyses can be used to identify the characteristics of an intervention that are most likely to result in the desired behavior change. Large effect sizes from a meta-analysis can then be combined with constructs from the social cognitive theory to design a more effective intervention, as was done in a study by Ransdell and colleagues (2003). More information about using effect sizes from meta-analyses to plan an intervention is included in the next section of this introduction.

Theories and models are also used to evaluate interventions. A physical activity intervention grounded in social cognitive theory can be compared to one that is not theory based to see which results in greater changes in physical activity or exercise participation and to discern which component of theory best predicted the behavior change of interest.

Finally, theories and models can be tested using a cross-sectional design. For example, people can be asked in a questionnaire which component of a specific theory would be most beneficial. Rather than address every aspect of a theory in a costly intervention, the most important factors can be delineated through a cross-sectional study, resulting in a more cost-effective intervention.

Use Effect Sizes From Meta-Analyses

Another important step when planning an intervention is to find a meta-analysis related to the type of intervention being planned. When human and financial resources are invested in a physical activity intervention, it is important to examine effect sizes from a meta-analysis—when available. Effect sizes give researchers a clear indication of the strength of a relationship between components of an intervention and any increases in physical activity. One of the most comprehensive meta-analytic studies ever completed on the topic of physical activity interventions was published by Dishman and Buckworth in 1996. Although this study is more than a decade old, it examined effect sizes in 127 studies with over 131,000 participants; no study this large has been completed since this one. The overall effect size for the success of physical activity interventions, corrected for sample size (e.g., large sample sizes were given more weight when the data from all studies were combined) was .34, which is considered moderate to large. Therefore, as professionals in the field, we can safely conclude that with appropriate planning and resources, physical activity interventions can be successful, especially over the short term.

The meta-analysis by Dishman and Buckworth (1996) also attempted to discern which components of a physical activity intervention were most predictive of changes in physical activity in a variety of populations. They concluded that three things were especially powerful in facilitating increases in physical activity: (a) the application of behavior modification principles such as increasing self-efficacy and using self-monitoring and positive self-talk, (b) the use of mediated delivery of information (e.g., Web-based or video), and (c) the prescription of low- to moderate-intensity physical activity. Behavior modification, mediated delivery, and activity intensity manipulation, as recommended for physical activity interventions, are covered in this book. Because other meta-analyses are available in a variety of areas, planners should check to see if one is available in their area of interest. This will allow them to use large effect sizes to ensure that the intervention will be successful.

Use Focus Groups

A final suggestion for anyone planning an intervention is to use focus groups to ascertain physical activity preferences and preferred intervention characteristics (e.g., the time and location of activities, types of activities, and instructor characteristics) (Gittlesohn et al., 2006). Focus groups are small groups of prospective participants who get together to discuss things that are important to them relative to the intervention. A facilitator usually leads the group through a series of questions designed to tease out important factors related to behavior change. If focus group information is collected from the target population (e.g., women or the elderly), it is more likely that people will feel invested in the program and participate in the program, and it is more likely that the intervention will be successful.

In conclusion, if intervention planners consider three basic steps prior to designing an intervention (i.e., establish a theoretical basis, use effect sizes, and use focus groups), it is likely that the intervention will result in a higher success rate compared to the one-size-fits-all approach.

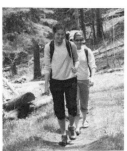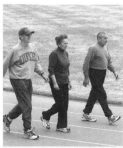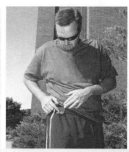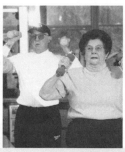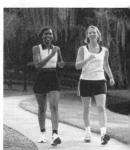

Thinking About the Foundations of Physical Activity

This part of the book provides important background information for physical activity researchers and practitioners. First, we include physical activity recommendations that were developed by federal agencies and professional organizations to promote and maintain health in adult populations. We also present an overview of scientific literature that is the foundation for the physical activity recommendations. Second, we give detailed information regarding the four cornerstones of physical activity promotion: needs assessment, program planning, program implementation, and program evaluation. Finally, we present information regarding techniques that can be used to measure physical activity and considerations when choosing a measurement technique. This part of the book is an invaluable resource because of the unique combination of material presented and resources provided.

PART

one

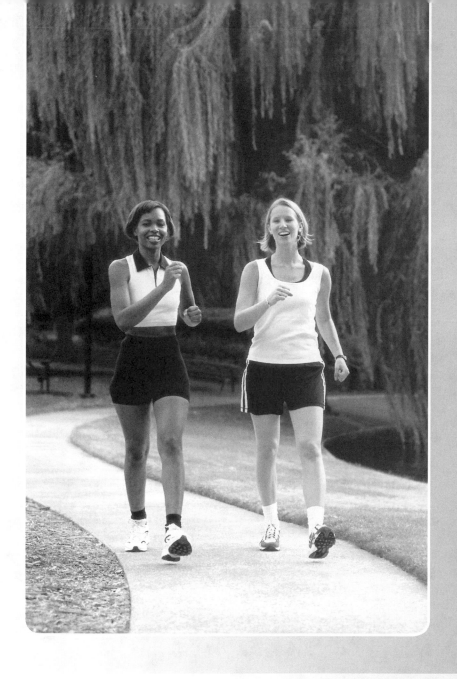

Promoting and Maintaining Health Through Physical Activity Recommendations

Physical inactivity is a major public health issue in the United States and in developed countries around the world. The majority of adults do not engage in the recommended amounts of physical activity, obesity is on the rise, and health care costs for diseases associated with a sedentary lifestyle continue to skyrocket. A variety of media outlets, including popular magazines and television, dispense advice regarding physical activity. Sifting through all of the information to determine how much activity is actually needed to improve or maintain health can be difficult. Fortunately, several U.S. federal agencies and professional organizations have thoroughly reviewed the scientific literature and released physical activity recommendations to promote and maintain health in adults. These are the recommendations that practitioners and researchers should consider when planning physical activity interventions and programs. This chapter provides a brief overview of the underlying principles of physical activity, presents several physical activity recommendations, and summarizes the scientific literature that is the foundation for the recommendations.

Principles of Physical Activity

To interpret the physical activity recommendations, one must understand the physical activity principles of *frequency, intensity, duration*, and *mode*. *Frequency* refers to how often a person engages in physical activity. *Intensity* refers to the effort or metabolic cost of the activity; *duration* is the amount of time spent in physical activity; and *mode* is the type of physical activity.

The recommendations presented in the following section were developed by experts who examined scientific literature and data to determine the amount of physical activity needed to promote and maintain health in adult populations. They used the physical activity principles of frequency, duration, and intensity to calculate the dose (volume) of physical activity needed for health benefits.

Physical Activity Recommendations

Table 1.1 presents an overview of several physical activity recommendations to promote and maintain health for adults. A detailed description of each recommendation follows. Readers interested in exercise recommendations to promote physical fitness should consult *ACSM's Guidelines for Exercise Testing and Prescription* (American College of Sports Medicine, 2006).

U.S. Centers for Disease Control and Prevention and the American College of Sports Medicine

The first recommendation to promote the physical activity–health paradigm was released in 1995 by the U.S. Centers for Disease Control and Prevention (CDC) and the American College of Sports Medicine (ACSM). Experts recommended that "every U.S. adult should accumulate 30 minutes or more of moderate-intensity physical activity on most, preferably all, days of the

TABLE 1.1   **Adult Physical Activity Recommendations to Promote and Maintain Health**

Recommendation	Frequency	Intensity	Duration
CDC/ACSM (Pate et al., 1995)	Most days of the week	Moderate (3-6 METs)	≥30 minutes/day
Surgeon general's report (U.S. Department of Health and Human Services, 1996)	Most days of the week	Moderate (3-6 METs)	≥30 minutes/day
Institute of Medicine (Institute of Medicine, 2005)	Daily	Moderate (3-6 METs)	≥60 minutes/day
Dietary Guidelines for Americans (U.S. Department of Health and Human Services and U.S. Department of Agriculture, 2005)	Most days of the week	Moderate (3-6 METs)	≥30 minutes/day
ACSM/AHA (Haskell et al., 2007)	Moderate (5 days/week) Vigorous (3 days/week)	Moderate (3-5.9 METs) Vigorous (≥6 METs)	Moderate (≥30 minutes/day) Vigorous (≥20 minutes/day)
Physical Activity Guidelines for Americans (U.S. Department of Health and Human Services, 2008)	Spread throughout the week	Moderate (3-5.9 METs) Vigorous (≥6 METs)	Moderate (≥150 minutes/week) Vigorous (≥75 minutes/week)

week" (Pate et al., 1995, p. 404). Unique aspects of the recommendation included allowance for the accumulation of physical activity in short, intermittent bouts and the promotion of moderate-intensity physical activity (3-6 METs). One MET is equal to the resting metabolic rate of a person, which is approximately 3.5 milliliters of oxygen per kilogram of body mass per minute (Kriska & Caspersen, 1997). Therefore, physical activities of 3 METs require energy expenditure three times the resting metabolic rate.

U.S. Surgeon General's Report on Physical Activity and Health

Physical Activity and Health: A Report of the Surgeon General was published in 1996 (U.S. Department of Health and Human Services, 1996). The U.S. surgeon general's recommendation reiterated the CDC/ACSM recommendation (Pate et al., 1995) to accumulate at least 30 minutes of moderate-intensity physical activity on most days of the week. In addition, the report stated that "activity leading to an increase in daily expenditure of approximately 150 kilocalories/day (equivalent to about 1,000 kilocalories/week) is associated with substantial health benefits and that the activity does not need to be vigorous to achieve benefit" (p. 147).

Institute of Medicine

The Institute of Medicine examined cross-sectional data to determine a recommended level of physical activity. Because 60 minutes of daily moderate-intensity physical activity or shorter periods of more vigorous exertion was associated with normal body mass index (BMI) values (18.5 to 25 kg/m²), the

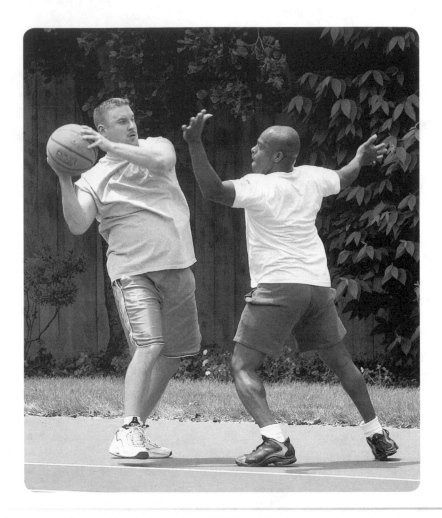

The American College of Sports Medicine (ACSM) and the American Heart Association (AHA) recommend that healthy adults engage in moderate-intensity aerobic physical activity for a minimum of 30 minutes on five days each week or vigorous-intensity aerobic activity for a minimum of 20 minutes on three days each week to promote and maintain health (Haskell et al., 2007).

Institute of Medicine recommended that amount of activity for normal-weight adults (Institute of Medicine, 2005). BMI is the ratio of weight to height and is typically calculated by dividing weight in kilograms by height in meters squared (kg/m^2) (American College of Sports Medicine, 2006). BMI values > 25 are associated with increased risk of chronic disease (American College of Sports Medicine, 2006).

Dietary Guidelines for Americans

The U.S. Department of Health and Human Services and the U.S. Department of Agriculture released the *Dietary Guidelines for Americans* in 2005. They recommended that adults engage in at least 30 minutes of moderate-intensity physical activity on most, but preferably all, days of the week to reduce the risk of chronic disease in adulthood. In addition, they recommended approximately 60 minutes of moderate- to vigorous-intensity activity to manage body weight and prevent the gradual accumulation of excess body weight in adulthood (U.S. Department of Health and Human Services & U.S. Department of Agriculture, 2005).

American College of Sports Medicine and the American Heart Association

An expert panel of scientists from the American College of Sports Medicine (ACSM) and the American Heart Association (AHA) reviewed the recent scientific literature to update the original CDC/ACSM recommendation that was published in 1995 (Pate et al., 1995). Their intention was "to provide a more comprehensive and explicit public health recommendation for adults based upon available evidence of the health benefits of physical activity" (Haskell et al., 2007, p. 1425). Their recommendation was "to promote and maintain health, all healthy adults aged 18-65 years need moderate intensity aerobic physical activity for a minimum of 30 minutes on five days each week or vigorous intensity aerobic activity for a minimum of 20 minutes on three days each week" (p. 1425). The recommended amount of aerobic activity is in addition to light-intensity routine activities of daily living or activities lasting less than 10 minutes. In addition, they stated that moderate and vigorous physical activity could be combined to meet the recommendation and that aerobic activity of at least moderate intensity could be accumulated toward the 30-minute daily minimum in bouts lasting at least 10 minutes. They also explicitly stated that participation in physical activity above the recommended amount provides additional health benefits and results in higher levels of physical fitness. Furthermore, they also emphasized the importance of muscular strength and endurance activities to promote and maintain health and recommended that "adults perform activities that maintain or increase muscular strength and endurance for a minimum of two days each week" (Haskell et al., 2007, p. 1426).

This recommendation clarified several issues from the CDC/ACSM recommendation (Pate et al., 1995). Aerobic (endurance) activity was specified, an exact frequency of activity was stated, accumulation was clarified, and both moderate- and vigorous-intensity physical activity were addressed.

Physical Activity Guidelines for Americans

The U.S. Department of Health and Human Services released the *2008 Physical Activity Guidelines for Americans* during the fall of 2008. For substantial health benefits, they recommended that adults engage in at least 150 minutes of moderate intensity, or 75 minutes of vigorous intensity, aerobic physical activity throughout the week. Furthermore, they suggested that aerobic activity be accumulated in bouts of at least 10 minutes; that the activity should be spread throughout the week, and that the moderate and vigorous intensity activities could be combined to meet the recommendation. They also emphasized that individuals could gain additional health benefits by increasing their weekly physical activity beyond the recommended amount stated above and by participating in muscle strengthening activities at least two or more days per week (U.S. Department of Health and Human Services, 2008).

Scientific Foundation for the Recommendations

Experts reviewed the scientific literature and data to determine the relationships among physical activity, mortality, and morbidity. In general, there is a large decrease in the risk of adverse health conditions when physical activity level increases from low to moderate, with a further but smaller decrease in risk when physical activity level moves from moderate to high (Institute of Medicine, 2007). "Regardless of the morbidity, mortality, or population group (with few exceptions), the evidence shows that those who are more physically active, get more exercise, or are more fit have lower risk" (Institute of Medicine, 2007, p. 142). The following sections summarize the relationships among physical activity, mortality, and major diseases. Readers who are interested in learning more about the associations between physical activity and a variety of chronic diseases should consult the special issue of *Medicine & Science in Sports & Exercise* (Kesaniemi et al., 2001) and *Physical Activity and Health* (Bouchard, Blair, & Haskell, 2007).

All-Cause Mortality

The first epidemiological studies to examine the relationship between physical activity and mortality were conducted on London busmen and postal workers by Professor Jeremy Morris and on San Francisco dockworkers and Harvard alumni by Professor Ralph Paffenbarger (Blair & LaMonte, 2007). Their studies "provided the first prospective, systematic examination of physical inactivity and adverse health effects" (Blair & LaMonte, 2007, p. 145). Collectively, the results of their studies showed that physical activity is an important and independent predictor of all-cause mortality.

Expert panels and comprehensive literature reviews have confirmed that there is an inverse, dose-response relationship between physical activity and all-cause mortality (Haskell et al., 2007; Lee & Skerrett, 2001; U.S. Department of Health and Human Services, 1996). A dose-response relationship indicates that a change in physical activity level is associated with a graded change in the health outcome (Blair & LaMonte, 2007).

The relationship between physical activity and all-cause mortality has been documented in men and women, and in younger and older adults (Lee & Skerrett, 2001). Expending approximately 1,000 kilocalories per week in physical activity decreases the risk of all-cause mortality by 20 to 30% (Lee & Skerrett, 2001).

Cardiovascular Disease

Cardiovascular disease (CVD) is the leading cause of death in the United States (Minino, Heron, Murphy, & Kochankek, 2007). CVD is an inclusive term that includes coronary heart disease (CHD), hypertension, stroke, peripheral vascular disease, and other conditions of the cardiovascular system. The results of numerous studies indicate that physical activity is inversely associated with CVD risk (Haskell et al., 2007; Kohl, 2001; U.S. Department of Health and Human Services, 1996), with significantly lower risks observed with as little as 45 minutes per week of brisk walking (Haskell et al., 2007).

The exact shape of the dose-response curve between physical activity and CVD may depend on the specific CVD outcome of interest and the baseline activity levels of the population (Haskell et al., 2007). For example, the dose-response relationship between coronary heart disease (CHD) and physical activity level appears to be inverse and curvilinear, suggesting that the largest reduction in CHD risk occurs when a sedentary person begins participating in moderate levels of physical activity (Janssen, 2007). Higher levels of physical activity provide additional protective effects, indicating that the most active individuals have the lowest risk of developing CHD (Haskell et al., 2007; Janssen, 2007). The relationship is evident in men and women and ethnically diverse populations (Haskell et al., 2007). The dose-response relationship between stroke and physical activity is less clear. The relationship may be U-shaped with increased risk of stroke for those who are inactive and those who are highly active (Kohl, 2001; U.S. Department of Health and Human Services, 1996), or the shape may be inverse and curvilinear, similar to the relationship between physical activity and CHD (Janssen, 2007).

Cancer

Cancer is the second leading cause of death in the United States (Minino et al., 2007). In 2004 approximately one out of every four deaths was attributable to cancer (Minino et al., 2007). Numerous studies have been conducted to determine the relationship between physical activity and several site-specific cancers (Thune & Furberg, 2001). To date, the strongest evidence indicates an inverse, dose-response relationship between physical activity and cancer of the colon and breast (Lee, 2007; Thune & Furberg, 2001). Additional research is needed to clarify the relationship between physical activity and other cancers.

Physically active people have a lower risk of developing colon cancer than their less active peers (Lee, 2007). The average reduction in colon cancer risk is approximately 30% among physically active men and women when compared to inactive people (Lee, 2007). Available information suggests that 30 to 45 minutes per day of moderate-intensity physical activity is sufficient to reduce risk (Lee, 2007). There are not enough data at this time to determine the additional protective effects of greater amounts of physical activity (Lee, 2007).

There is an inverse, dose-response relationship between physical activity and breast cancer in women (Lee, 2007; Thune & Furberg, 2001). Lee (2007) examined the results from numerous studies and determined that, on average, active women had a 20% lower risk of developing breast cancer than their less active peers. It appears that "4 to 7 hr/week of moderate- to vigorous-intensity physical activity is required" (p. 212) to decrease the risk of breast cancer (Lee, 2007). Similar to colon cancer, there is currently not enough information to indicate how much physical activity is needed to observe greater reductions in breast cancer risk (Lee, 2007).

Type 2 Diabetes Mellitus

Diabetes is the most common type of endocrine disorder and is the sixth leading cause of death in the United States (Minino et al., 2007). Type 2 diabetes is frequently linked to obesity and is characterized as a metabolic disorder in which insulin levels are typically elevated (Alcazar, Ho, & Goodyear, 2007). Regular physical activity can prevent or delay the onset of type 2 diabetes (Alcazar et al., 2007; Kelley & Goodpaster, 2001) irrespective of ethnicity, gender, or age group (Alcazar et al., 2007). Experts examined data from several large-scale studies and concluded that approximately 30 minutes of moderate-intensity physical activity at least 5 days per week provides a 25 to 36% reduction in the risk of type 2 diabetes (Institute of Medicine, 2007).

Osteoporosis

Osteoporosis is a disease characterized by low bone mass and the deterioration of bone tissue (Vuori, 2001) and is commonly defined by bone mineral density (BMD). BMD 2.5 standard deviations or more below the young adult mean is indicative of osteoporosis (Vuori, 2001).

Physical activity may affect BMD at three time periods during a lifetime: (a) During childhood and adolescence, weight-bearing activity helps to develop peak bone mass, (b) during the second through fifth decades, physical activity helps to maintain peak bone mass, and (c) later in adult life physical activity slows the rate of BMD decline as much as 1% per year (Hootman, 2007). "Moderate to strong evidence indicates that physical activity plays an important role in optimizing bone health during the developmental years; but the long-term effects are not well known, and dose-response information is lacking" (Institute of Medicine, 2007, p. 26).

Mental Health

Physical activity can provide psychological benefits for healthy people as well as those suffering from mild to moderate emotional illnesses (Raglin, Wilson, & Galper, 2007; U.S. Department of Health and Human Services, 1996). The most commonly studied mental health conditions are anxiety disorders and depression.

Anxiety disorders are the most common form of emotional illness, with about 17% of U.S. adults seeking treatment annually (Raglin et al., 2007). In the epidemiological literature, physical activity is consistently associated with fewer symptoms of anxiety, and the odds of anxiety symptoms are reduced by 25 to 50% (Institute of Medicine, 2007). Additional research is needed to determine the dose-response relationship between physical activity and anxiety disorders (Dunn, Trivedi, & O'Neal, 2001; Institute of Medicine, 2007; Raglin et al., 2007).

Another common mental disorder is depression. Depression will afflict one out of three people in the United States during their lives (Raglin et al., 2007). There is consistent evidence that physical activity is associated with reduced symptoms of depression (Dunn et al., 2001; Institute of Medicine, 2007). Physically active people have a 30 to 50% reduction in the odds of depression symptoms (Institute of Medicine, 2007). Although a dose-response relationship between physical activity and depression is plausible, additional research is needed to determine the association (Dunn et al., 2001; Institute of Medicine, 2007; Raglin et al., 2007).

❑ Understand the principles of physical activity including frequency, intensity, duration, and mode.

❑ Determine the dose of physical activity needed to promote and maintain health for the target population by reviewing the recommendations issued by federal agencies and professional organizations.

❑ Become familiar with the relationship between physical activity and specific diseases by reviewing the scientific literature.

GETTING STARTED

Summary

Physical inactivity is a major public health issue in the United States and abroad. Because regular physical activity conveys numerous health benefits, several professional organizations and U.S. government agencies have issued physical activity recommendations for adults to improve or maintain health. The recommendations are based on the results from scientific studies that have examined the relationship between physical activity and a variety of health outcomes. The unequivocal evidence of a dose-response relationship between physical activity and all-cause mortality, cardiovascular disease, colon and breast cancer, and type 2 diabetes mellitus provides the foundation for the recommendations.

The majority of recommendations presented in this chapter encourage adults to participate in 30 minutes or more of moderate-intensity physical activity at least 5 days per week. In addition, recent recommendations explicitly state that additional health benefits may be obtained by engaging in additional physical activity beyond the minimum recommended amount. Developers of physical activity interventions should consider the individual and group goals of participants, program resources, and facilities, in conjunction with the scientific evidence to use the most effective physical activity recommendation possible. Strategies presented throughout this book will enable physical activity program developers to design effective programs with measurable and realistic outcomes.

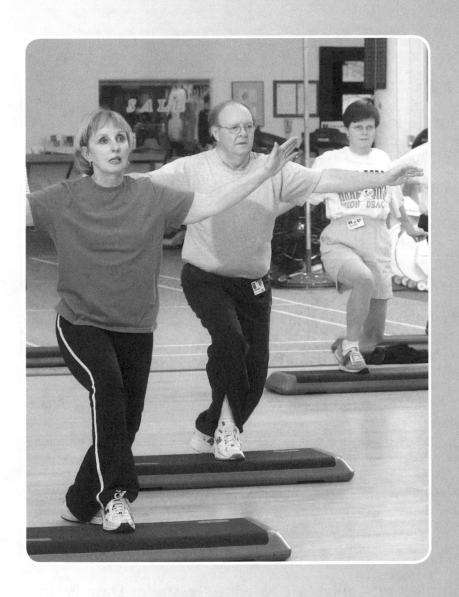

CHAPTER 2

Planning and Evaluating Physical Activity Programs

Four cornerstones provide the foundation of physical activity promotion: needs assessment, program planning, program implementation, and program evaluation. Briefly, needs assessment involves determining the physical activity–related needs of the target population; program planning involves developing the program; program implementation involves delivering the program to the target population; and program evaluation involves assessing the program to determine its effectiveness. This chapter presents an overview of the four cornerstones of physical activity promotion. Additional planning and evaluation resources are also included.

Program Needs

A physical activity program should not be initiated without first conducting a needs assessment. The purpose of the needs assessment is to determine the specific physical activity–related needs of the target population. During this phase, it is extremely important to collect primary data from members of the target population, as well as to examine secondary data sources (McKenzie, Neiger, & Smeltzer, 2005).

Physical activity professionals need to interact with, and collect data from, members of the target population to determine their perceived needs. Focus groups, community forums, interviews, and surveys are some of the techniques that can be used to do this. Physical activity professionals may want to use several of the techniques to obtain a comprehensive picture of the target population's needs. When deciding which of the techniques to use, the physical activity professional should consider the type and amount of information needed, the available resources, and the target population. For example, a survey administered through intraoffice mail may work well in a worksite setting. However, a community forum or focus groups may be best to determine the needs of a larger community. These techniques are briefly described in the following text.

Techniques for Collecting Needs Assessment Data From the Target Population

Focus Groups

- 8-12 members of the target population
- Predetermined questions are asked by a trained facilitator
- Participant responses are audio or video recorded
- Transcripts are generated
- Transcripts are analyzed for patterns to determine needs

Nominal Group Process

- 5-7 knowledgeable representatives from the target population

- Individuals record their own responses and then share their responses with the group
- Individual responses are recorded by the facilitator for all to see and hear
- Group members prioritize the items on the list that was generated from individual responses
- Group agrees on final ranking of needs

Community Forum

- Large gathering of target population members
- Moderator asks those present to share their concerns and express the physical activity needs of the target population
- The session may be audio or video recorded
- Participants may also be asked to respond in writing
- Notes, transcripts, and data are analyzed to determine needs

Interviews

- Members of the target population are individually interviewed to determine their perceptions regarding the physical activity needs of the target population
- Trained interviewer asks a set of questions
- Session is typically audio recorded
- Transcripts are generated and analyzed to determine needs

Surveys

- Typically written questionnaires
- Questionnaires can be administered face-to-face, through the mail, over the telephone, or via the Internet
- Member of the target population or opinion leaders may be surveyed
- Data are compiled and analyzed to determine needs

Observation

- Observing behavior in the appropriate setting
- Walking/bicycle trail use, recreational facilities use, etc.
- Data are analyzed to determine needs

From McKenzie et al. 2005.

Physical activity professionals should also use secondary sources such as reports, scientific literature, and data sets to help determine the needs of the target population. For example, federal documents such as *Healthy People 2010* (U.S. Department of Health and Human Services, 2000) and national databases such as National Health and Nutrition Examination Survey (NHANES) data (Centers for Disease Control and Prevention, 2007b) are excellent sources.

Furthermore, state and local health department reports, as well as Behavior Risk Factor Surveillance System (BRFSS) data (Centers for Disease Control and Prevention, 2007a), are very useful.

Once data have been collected from the target population and secondary sources of information have been gathered, the next step is to assess and synthesize all of the information to determine the focus of the program to be developed. Priority should always be given to important needs that can be met (Green & Kreuter, 2005).

Program Planning

When the physical activity–related needs of the target population have been determined, the planning phase begins. Program stakeholders, those with a vested interest in the program, should be identified and involved in all aspects of the planning phase. During this phase, program developers identify potential program partners, develop goals and objectives, determine specific intervention activities, and verify resources.

Identifying Potential Program Partners

Potential program partners may be financial supporters, sponsors, agencies or organizations, and previously identified stakeholders. Physical activity professionals should identify potential program partners early so they can offer input during the planning phase. *Promoting Physical Activity: A Guide for Community Action* (U.S. Department of Health and Human Services, 1999) is an excellent resource that contains an entire chapter on identifying and working with partners.

Developing Goals and Objectives

Goals are general statements about what the program intends to accomplish. Goals are usually not directly measurable. Goal statements should contain *who* and *what*. Objectives are specific, measurable steps toward a goal. Objectives should contain the *outcome, condition, criteria*, and *target population* (McKenzie et al., 2005). Objectives should also be SMART: specific, measurable, achievable, relevant, and time bound (U.S. Department of Health and Human Services, 2002). Sample goals and objectives from *Healthy People 2010* (U.S. Department of Health and Human Services, 2000) are presented in the following text.

Physical Activity Goal and Objectives from *Healthy People 2010*

Healthy People 2010 Physical Activity Goal

Improve health, fitness, and quality of life of Americans through daily physical activity
Who: Americans
What: Improve health, fitness, and quality of life

Healthy People 2010 Objective 22-2

Increase the proportion of adults who engage regularly, preferably daily, in moderate physical activity for at least 30 minutes per day from 15% to 30% by 2010.
Outcome (what): Increase daily moderate physical activity
Condition (when): By 2010
Criteria (how much): To 30%
Target population (who): Adults

Healthy People 2010 Objective 22-3

Increase the proportion of adults who engage in vigorous physical activity that promotes the development and maintenance of cardiorespiratory fitness 3 or more days per week for 20 or more minutes per occasion from 23% to 30% by 2010.
Outcome (what): Increase vigorous physical activity
Condition (when): By 2010
Criteria (how much): To 30%
Target population (who): Adults

From McKenzie et al., 2005; U.S. Department of Health and Human Services, 2000.

Developing Intervention Activities

When deciding which specific activities to incorporate in the intervention, planners should select activities that are based on appropriate behavior change theories or models and are suitable for the target population. Ideally, the strategies that are incorporated into the intervention will have documented effectiveness in a population similar to the target population.

The Task Force on Community Preventive Services systematically reviewed and evaluated numerous physical activity studies to determine intervention effectiveness (Centers for Disease Control and Prevention, 2001; Task Force on Community Preventive Services, 2005). They examined three categories of physical activity interventions: informational, behavioral and social, and environmental and policy. Several intervention approaches were recommended based on the evidence compiled. Those recommendations are briefly described in the following sections. In addition, informational interventions and behavioral and social interventions are described in chapters 4 through 7. Chapter 8 presents environmental and policy approaches.

Informational Approaches Informational interventions include educational activities to enhance participants' knowledge of physical activity, increase awareness, and provide motivation for participants to become more physically active. Recommended approaches within this category include community-wide campaigns and point-of-decision prompts to encourage stair use.

Community-wide campaigns are large-scale, broad-based interventions that use numerous media outlets to deliver the intervention message. In addition, these interventions may include risk factor screening at various locations within the community, widely available physical activity counseling, support groups, community-wide events, and the creation of walking trails. Point-of-decision prompts are signs placed near elevators and escalators to encourage the use of stairs. The messages on the signs should be adapted to the target population.

Behavioral and Social Approaches   Behavioral and social interventions involve enhancing behavior management skills and creating a social environment that is conducive to increasing physical activity. These interventions may include teaching skills pertaining to planning for physical activity, recognizing high-risk situations, and preventing relapse. They may also involve changing the work or home environment to support physical activity. Recommended approaches within this category that target adult populations include social support interventions in community settings and individually adapted behavior change programs.

Social support interventions focus on building and enhancing social support networks that encourage physical activity. Families, worksites, and entire communities may be involved. Individually adapted behavior change programs are tailored to people's interests, readiness to change, and skill level. Activities may focus on goal setting, positive self-talk, and problem solving. Established health behavior change models provide the foundation of these interventions.

Environmental and Policy Approaches   These interventions involve changing the physical environment, norms, policies, and laws of a community. The Task Force on Community Preventive Services (2005) recommended

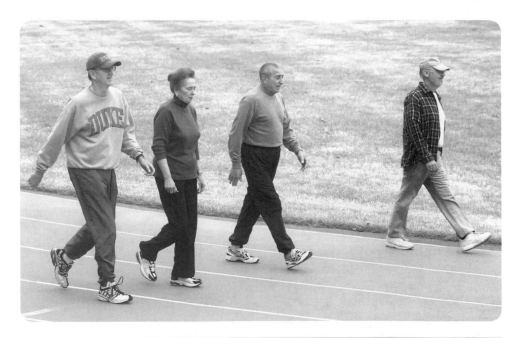

Improving and maintaining access to local physical activity facilities is an important environmental and policy approach for physical activity promotion professionals to consider because it provides community members the opportunity to be physically active.

approaches to create or improve access to places for physical activity. Examples include creating walking trails, building exercise facilities, and providing or increasing access to existing facilities. In addition, the Task Force recommended community and street-scale urban design and land use policies for increasing physical activity. Additional information is available at www.thecommunityguide.org/pa/ (Centers for Disease Control and Prevention, 2006).

Verifying Adequate Resources for the Program

As the planning phase is nearing completion, physical activity professionals should make certain that adequate resources are available for the program they are planning. This phase may take a considerable amount of time and effort depending on the stage of the program. For example, a new program will require much more time because qualified staff may need to be recruited, materials may need to be ordered, and facilities may need to be identified. However, an ongoing program that is being revised may require less effort at this stage because the staff and materials are already available. Professionals need to make sure that funding for the program has been secured, qualified staff have been hired, access to the necessary facilities is available, and equipment and materials are available or have been ordered before the program is implemented.

Program Implementation

The third cornerstone of physical activity promotion is program implementation. During this phase, the program is marketed, participants are recruited, and the program begins. Safety of participants and staff should always be a priority. Competent, trained staff should conduct the intervention activities. In addition, physical activity professionals should offer program activities in safe locations and keep all equipment in working order. An emergency action plan and safety manual should be developed, and all staff should be trained in emergency procedures. Furthermore, informed consent should be obtained from all program participants.

Newly developed interventions should be pilot tested if possible. This involves initially offering a smaller version of the intervention to a smaller group of people. During the pilot test, the physical activity professional should elicit feedback from participants and observe the intervention activities in order to revise and refine the intervention.

To recruit participants, planners should advertise the intervention to members of the target population. There are many places to advertise the program including newsletters, posters, brochures, bulletin boards, billboards, e-mail, payroll stuffers, newspapers, and television (Anspaugh, Dignan, & Anspaugh, 2006). In addition, personal interaction and announcements at group meetings may be effective—especially if done by members of the target population. It is important that planners use advertising techniques that will reach the desired target population. For example, a newspaper advertisement will reach a different segment of the target population than will an advertisement placed on a social Web site.

Program Evaluation

The fourth cornerstone of physical activity promotion is evaluation. Although it is the final cornerstone, evaluation of the program should not be an after-thought. The evaluation plan should be considered and developed throughout the planning process. During the evaluation process, physical activity professionals should collect the data needed to determine whether program objectives were achieved. An excellent resource is the *Physical Activity Evaluation Handbook,* which is available at www.cdc.gov/nccdphp/dnpa (U.S. Department of Health and Human Services, 2002).

There are three types of evaluation: process, impact, and outcome (Green & Lewis, 1986). Process evaluation is a type of formative evaluation that occurs as the program is being developed and implemented. Impact evaluation is a type of summative evaluation that is conducted at or near the end of the program to determine the actual impact of the program. Outcome evaluation is another type of summative evaluation that involves following participants for months or perhaps years to assess long-term changes (Green & Lewis, 1986). Sample process, impact, and outcome evaluation questions for a physical activity program are presented in the following text.

Sample Evaluation Questions for a Physical Activity Intervention

Process Evaluation

- Is the program being delivered as planned?
- Are participants attending program activities and events?
- Are external factors affecting the program?
- Are we reaching the target population?
- What is working well? Why?
- What is not working well? Why?
- Should we change the time or location of the program (or both)?

Impact Evaluation

- Did participants increase their physical activity?
- Did participants enjoy the program?
- Are participants meeting current physical activity recommendations?
- How expensive was the program?
- Did participants improve their physical fitness?

Outcome Evaluation

- How many participants remain physically active 6 months after the program? 12 months after the program? 18 to 24 months after the program?
- Has prevalence of physical inactivity decreased in the community?

During the evaluation phase, physical activity professionals should determine the specific data that they will need to collect to determine whether the program was successful. Each objective that was developed in the program planning phase should be evaluated. At a minimum, process and impact evaluation should be conducted, with outcome evaluation added as the program matures. An evaluation design should be selected that allows for the most rigorous evaluation possible while considering the available resources, staff expertise, time line, and participant burden (U.S. Department of Health and Human Services, 2002).

❑ Identify specific physical activity–related needs of the target population.
❑ Consider both primary and secondary data when determining needs.
❑ Identify program partners early in the planning process.
❑ Determine the goals and objectives of the program.
❑ Use intervention activities that are based on appropriate behavior change theories or models and are suitable for the target population.
❑ Incorporate into the intervention the strategies that have documented effectiveness in a population similar to the target population.
❑ Implement the program once adequate resources have been secured.
❑ Consider process, impact, and outcome evaluation.

GETTING STARTED

Summary

The four cornerstones of physical activity promotion are needs assessment, program development, program implementation, and program evaluation. A comprehensive needs assessment should be conducted prior to planning a physical activity program. Physical activity professionals should use the needs assessment data to determine the focus of the program. Goals and objectives should be developed, and theoretically based intervention activities that are appropriate for the target population should be planned. Safety should be a priority when implementing the program, and a comprehensive evaluation should be conducted to determine program effectiveness.

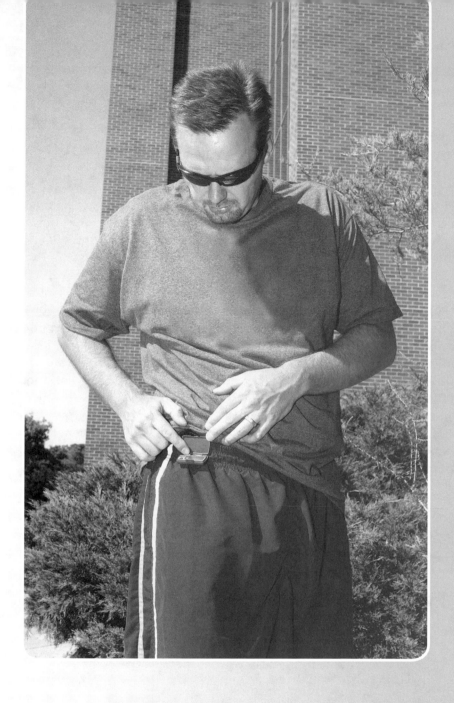

CHAPTER 3

Measuring
Physical Activity

Physical activity is any bodily movement that results in energy expenditure (Caspersen, Powell, & Christenson, 1985). It is a behavior—something a person does. Physical activity can occur at work (taking the stairs instead of the elevator), around the home or yard (sweeping, mowing, raking), during leisure time (jogging, golf), and for transportation (walking to the store, bicycling to work). People may engage in physical activity throughout the day in short bouts, or they may participate in longer bouts of physical activity for exercise. Because physical activity can occur in a variety of settings and formats, it can be difficult to accurately assess a person's participation in physical activity.

Physical fitness, which is a characteristic a person may possess as a result of participation in physical activity or exercise, can be an indicator of physical activity participation. Researchers and practitioners should consider the goals of their interventions to determine what specific health or fitness outcomes to assess. If the intervention is designed to increase physical activity to a level that should elicit gains in physical fitness, then fitness components should be measured as outcomes. However, because all physical activity does not result in fitness improvement, physical activity should always be assessed as an outcome measure of any physical activity intervention.

Direct measures of physical activity reflect actual bodily movement or energy expenditure, whereas indirect measures are surrogate markers of physical activity (Ainsworth, 2000b). Several direct and indirect measures

TABLE 3.1   Physical Activity Measures and Their Advantages and Disadvantages

Type of measurement	Advantages	Disadvantages
Questionnaire	• Inexpensive • Simple • Unobtrusive • Low participant burden • Can easily be used in large studies	• Dependence on recall • Lack of precision • Overestimation of physical activity • Social desirability
Pedometer	• Relatively inexpensive • Objective • Easy to use	• Cannot identify specific activities • No measure of intensity • Participant compliance may be an issue
Accelerometer	• Objective • Captures intensity of movement • Can examine patterns of activity	• Expensive • Waist-worn device captures ambulatory activity only • Participant compliance may be an issue • Data management issues

are available to assess physical activity in adult populations, including direct observation, physiological monitors, motion sensors, and questionnaires. We have included information regarding questionnaires because they are the most commonly used indirect measure, and motion sensors (pedometers and accelerometers) because they are becoming popular as direct measures of physical activity. Table 3.1 lists the advantages and disadvantages of the three measures. The following sections provide an overview of these methods of measuring physical activity in adults.

Physical Activity Questionnaires

Questionnaires can be interviewer- or self-administered and require that participants self-report their participation in physical activity over a specified time frame. Questionnaires may be classified as global, historical, or recall surveys depending on the time frame of recall and the information requested (Ainsworth, 2000b). *Global surveys* inquire about respondents' general physical activity habits and typically consist of three to five items. These questionnaires are easy to administer and do not place much of a burden on participants because they typically take approximately 5 minutes to complete. *Historical questionnaires* are detailed accounts of participants' physical activity frequency, intensity, and duration. The time frame of recall can range from the past year to a lifetime. Historical questionnaires provide a comprehensive picture of a person's physical activity participation and can allow for the examination of seasonal effects. However, they are very cumbersome to complete and may be limited by people's inability to remember their participation in physical activity over very long periods of time. *Recall questionnaires* ask about physical activity completed during the past week to past month. They typically have 10 to 30 items and allow for the calculation of energy expended in various intensities of physical activity (Ainsworth, 2000b). These questionnaires are fairly easy to complete, but they are limited to represent only the time frame of recall (1 to 4 weeks). There are many global, historical, and recall physical activity questionnaires from which to choose. A brief listing of questionnaires within each classification category is included in the following text.

Physical Activity Questionnaires

Global

- Godin Leisure-Time (Godin & Shephard, 1985)
- Health Insurance Plan of New York (HIP) (Shapiro, Weinblatt, Frank, & Sager, 1969)
- Lipid Research Clinics (Ainsworth, Jacobs, & Leon, 1993)
- Stanford Usual Activity (Sallis et al., 1985)

Historical

- CARDIA Physical Activity History (Jacobs, Hahn, Haskell, Pirie, & Sidney, 1989)
- Historical Leisure Activity (Kriska et al., 1990)
- Minnesota Leisure-Time (Taylor et al., 1978)
- Tecumseh Occupational (Montoye, 1971)

Recall

- 7-Day Physical Activity Recall (Sallis et al., 1985)
- Baecke (Baecke, Burema, & Frijters, 1982)
- Physical Activity Scale for the Elderly (Washburn, Smith, Jette, & Janney, 1993)
- International Physical Activity Questionnaire (IPAQ) (Craig et al., 2003)

When selecting a questionnaire, researchers and practitioners should consider the amount of information desired, the domain(s) of physical activity to assess, the preferred method of administration for the survey, the validity and reliability of the instrument, and the population to be surveyed. It is vitally important to make sure that the instrument is appropriate for the target population (item type, specific physical activities requested, reading level, etc.). The items included on the questionnaire should reflect activities that are suitable for members of the target population. "Older women, especially minority women, perform little structured sports and exercise activities. Instead, moderate-intensity activities related to the care of the home, family, and occupation make up much of the physical activity obtained during the day" (Ainsworth, 2000a, p. 96). Therefore, researchers and practitioners who are interested in assessing physical activity in older women should seek out valid questionnaires that inquire about moderate-intensity physical activities across the various domains of physical activity. Sallis and Saelens (2000) offer more information about the validity and reliability of various questionnaires.

Two types of data can be obtained from questionnaires: (a) time spent in physical activity and (b) energy expenditure (Kriska & Caspersen, 1997). Total time spent in physical activity is determined by multiplying the frequency of the activity by the duration of each activity session. An estimate of energy expenditure (MET hours per week) can be determined by multiplying the average hours per week of physical activity by the average intensity of the activity, expressed as metabolic equivalents (METs). As mentioned in chapter 1, 1 MET is equal to the resting metabolic rate of a person, which is approximately 3.5 milliliters of oxygen per kilogram of body mass per minute, or approximately 1 kilocalorie per kilogram of body mass per hour (Kriska & Caspersen, 1997). Therefore, physical activities of 4 METs require energy expenditure four times the resting metabolic rate. The MET values for numerous activities are available in the "Compendium of Physical Activities" (Ainsworth, Haskell, et al., 2000). Activities requiring 3.0 to 5.99 METs are of moderate intensity, whereas activities requiring at least 6.0 METS are categorized as being of vigorous intensity (Pate et al., 1995). For example, a person reports jogging 3 times per week for 30 minutes per session. This person spends 90 minutes a week (3 times/week $\times$ 30 minutes/session = 90 minutes/week), or 1.5 hours per week jogging. According to the "Compendium of Physical Activities," jogging is a 7 MET activity (Ainsworth, Haskell, et al., 2000). Therefore, the energy expenditure for this person is 10.5 MET-hours per week.

We present detailed information on a few frequently used physical activity questionnaires in the following sections. Readers who are interested in viewing samples of physical activity questionnaires should consult the collection of physical activity questionnaires that was published as a special issue of *Medicine & Science in Sports & Exercise* in 1997 (Kriska & Caspersen, 1997). Although published more than a decade ago, this supplement is an excellent resource to help with questionnaire selection.

Godin Leisure-Time Exercise Questionnaire

The Godin Leisure-Time Exercise Questionnaire (Godin & Shephard, 1985) is a global survey. When completing the survey, participants are asked to consider a 7-day period and report the average number of times they engage in physical activity for more than 15 minutes during their free time. The questionnaire contains two items. The first item requires participants to report their frequency of strenuous, moderate, and mild activity. The second item asks participants to report how frequently during the same week they participated in activity long enough to work up a sweat. Reported frequencies of strenuous, moderate, and light activities are multiplied by 9, 5, and 3 METs, respectively. Total weekly leisure activity is determined by summing the products of the three intensity categories.

Minnesota Leisure-Time Physical Activity Questionnaire

The Minnesota Leisure-Time Physical Activity Questionnaire is a historical survey that requires participants to recall their participation in leisure-time physical activities during the previous 12 months (Taylor et al., 1978). Participants read through a list of 63 sports and recreational, yard, and household activities and check either *Yes* or *No* for each activity, depending on whether they participated in the activity during the last 12 months. For each activity checked *Yes*, participants report the specific months they engaged in the activity and the frequency and duration of their participation. For each activity, the product of intensity code, duration, frequency per month, and months per year is calculated and divided by 52 to determine the weekly activity metabolic index (AMI) units. AMI units are summed across all reported activities to determine the total weekly AMI.

Seven-Day Physical Activity Recall

The Seven-Day Physical Activity Recall (7DPAR) (Sallis et al., 1985) is a recall survey. Participants report all moderate, hard, and very hard physical activities completed during the morning, afternoon, and evening on each of the previous 7 days. Participants also record the number of hours they slept during each 24-hour period. In addition, they report their employment status and the number of days and hours they worked during the past 7 days. They also identify what 2 days during the previous week they consider weekend days and compare their physical activity during the previous week to that of the previous 3 months. The number of hours spent in sleep and moderate, hard, and very hard activities are multiplied by their respective MET values and then summed across the categories to determine the total weekly energy expenditure.

Motion Sensors

Recently, pedometers and accelerometers have become popular because they provide an objective measure of physical activity, thereby alleviating some of the limitations of questionnaires. However, there are disadvantages to using pedometers and accelerometers (see table 3.1 on page 24). In the following sections we describe the monitors and provide a brief overview of issues to consider when using pedometers and accelerometers to assess physical activity.

Pedometers

Pedometers are small monitors that count the number of steps taken. They are user-friendly with easy-to-understand data output (i.e., steps). Furthermore, they allow for the objective and reliable measurement of ambulatory physical activity (Bassett, 2000) and are relatively inexpensive. Pedometers have been used to measure physical activity in epidemiological studies (Bassett, Schneider, & Huntington, 2004; Sequeira, Rickenbach, Wietlisbach, Tullen, & Schutz, 1995; Tudor-Locke et al., 2004) and are increasingly being used as self-monitoring tools in physical activity interventions (Dinger, Heesch, & McClary, 2005; DuVall et al., 2004; Tudor-Locke et al., 2002; Wilde, Sidman, & Corbin, 2001).

Many makes and models of pedometers are available. In addition to steps, some models estimate distance and caloric expenditure. Practitioners and researchers should use accurate pedometers to ensure that the step data they collect are a valid representation of their participants' ambulatory activity. The most accurate pedometers for counting steps in laboratory and field settings include the Yamax Digiwalker (SW-200, SW-701; $17-$30), Kenz Lifecorder ($200), and New Lifestyles NL-2000 ($60) (Crouter, Schneider, Karabulut, & Bassett, 2003; Schneider, Crouter, & Bassett, 2004). Most companies that sell pedometers provide a volume discount if numerous devices are purchased at one time.

Researchers and practitioners must consider several issues when using pedometers to measure ambulatory physical activity, including the data to report (steps, distance, or energy expenditure), the number of days to monitor participants, the data recording method, data collection, participant compliance, and reactivity (i.e., changing behavior because of monitoring). Researchers suggest reporting pedometer data as steps per day because this eliminates the need to adjust for height or body weight (Crouter et al., 2003; Schneider et al., 2004; Tudor-Locke & Myers, 2001). In addition, pedometers that count steps only are less expensive than those that report distance or energy expenditure, or both. Healthy younger adults accumulate 7,000 to 13,000 steps per day, whereas older adults accumulate 6,000 to 8,500 steps per day (Tudor-Locke & Myers, 2001). Step indices have been developed to aid in the interpretation of steps per day (Tudor-Locke & Bassett, 2004):

Number of Steps	Category
< 5,000	Sedentary
5,000-7,499	Low active
7,500-9,999	Somewhat active
10,000-12,499	Active
≥ 12,500	Highly active

Furthermore, reactivity to a pedometer does not appear to be a major threat to validity in adults (Behrens & Dinger, 2007; Matevey, Rogers, Dawson, & Tudor-Locke, 2006). Additional detailed information regarding methodological considerations when using pedometers is available elsewhere (Tudor-Locke & Myers, 2001).

Accelerometers

Accelerometers are small, pager-sized monitors that detect motion in one or more planes of movement. They are typically worn on a belt at the waist, over the right hip. The raw data from accelerometers are "counts." A count represents the intensity of movement and is actually the summation of the acceleration signals for the desired time period (i.e., a cycle). The data are stored by the accelerometers and downloaded to a computer for analysis. Accelerometers have been used to measure and describe physical activity in adults (Ainsworth, Bassett, et al., 2000; Buchowski, Acra, Majchrzak, Sun, & Chen, 2004; Dinger & Behrens, 2006; Matthews, Ainsworth, Thompson, & Bassett, 2002) and to assess intervention outcomes (DuVall et al., 2004). Accelerometers were also used to collect physical activity data from approximately 7,000 participants as part of the 2003-2004 National Health and Nutrition Examination Survey (Troiano, 2005).

Several makes and models of accelerometers are available. The ActiGraph (ActiGraph, LLC, Pensacola, FL) and RT3 Tri-axial Research Tracker (formerly Tritrac-R3D; Stayhealthy, Inc., Monrovia, CA) are the most commonly used

LIVERPOOL JOHN MOORES UNIVERSITY
LEARNING SERVICES

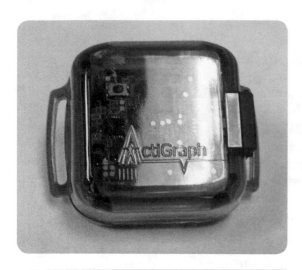

Accelerometers, like the ActiGraph GT1M, can be used to objectively measure physical activity.

uniaxial and triaxial accelerometers, respectively. Detailed information regarding commercially available accelerometers is available elsewhere (Trost, McIver, & Pate, 2005).

There are several issues to consider when using accelerometers to measure ambulatory physical activity in adults, including selecting an accelerometer, cycle length, the number of days to monitor, the distribution and collection of the devices, participant compliance, data management issues, and reactivity (Trost et al., 2005). Although 1-minute cycles have typically been used when assessing physical activity in adults (Buchowski et al., 2004; Dinger & Behrens, 2006; Matthews et al., 2002; Trost et al., 2005; Ward, Evenson, Vaughn, Rodgers, & Troiano, 2005), researchers recently have suggested using 10-second cycles (Crouter, Clowers, & Bassett, 2006). Although using the 10-second cycle length results in additional data to manage and analyze, it allows practitioners and researchers to distinguish among walking, running, and other activities, and it improves the prediction of energy expenditure (Crouter et al., 2006). Further, results of a recent study suggest that reactivity is not a serious threat to internal validity when using an accelerometer to assess physical activity in adults (Behrens & Dinger, 2007). Methodological considerations and best practices for using accelerometers have been published elsewhere (Trost et al., 2005; Ward et al., 2005).

GETTING STARTED

❑ Understand physical activity is a behavior that can be difficult to measure accurately.

❑ Consider the goals of interventions to determine the specific health or fitness outcomes to assess.

❑ Always assess physical activity as an outcome measure of any physical activity intervention.

❑ Use questionnaires to allow participants to self-report their physical activity.

❑ Ensure the questionnaire used is appropriate for the target population.

❑ Consider pedometers; they are small monitors that count the number of steps taken.

❑ Consider accelerometers, which are small monitors that detect motion in one or more planes of movement.

Summary

Although physical activity can be difficult to assess, researchers and practitioners should measure physical activity behavior when evaluating their interventions. Questionnaires are commonly used indirect measures of physical activity, whereas pedometers and accelerometers are direct measures that objectively assess physical activity by detecting actual bodily movement. Those interested in assessing physical activity should consider the advantages and disadvantages of each measure, as well as the issues highlighted in this chapter, when deciding what measurement technique to employ.

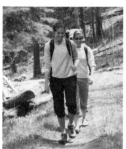
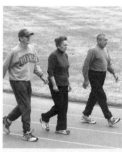
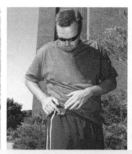
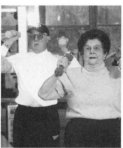
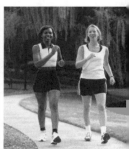

Working With Specific Populations

Understanding how to work with specific populations is of utmost importance to the success of physical activity interventions. For this reason, this part of the book provides information about working with specific populations. Women are less likely than men to be active and face unique barriers to physical activity. Chapter 4 includes ideas for designing programs that overcome those barriers. Chapter 5 addresses the factors related to successful interventions with overweight and obese populations as well as the common barriers people in these populations face. Chapter 6 addresses physical activity programs for older adults. Physical activity researchers and practitioners need to pay special attention to factors associated with physical activity in older adults considering that those who are 65 years and older are the fastest-growing population currently. Finally, those who have the highest rates of inactivity in the United States are those of ethnic diversity. Therefore, chapter 7 addresses the importance of cultural relevancy when designing physical activity intervention for ethnically diverse populations, as well as the strategies for overcoming the barriers these people face. Part II offers a wealth of information that will enable program designers and planners to create successful physical activity interventions for specific populations.

PART

two

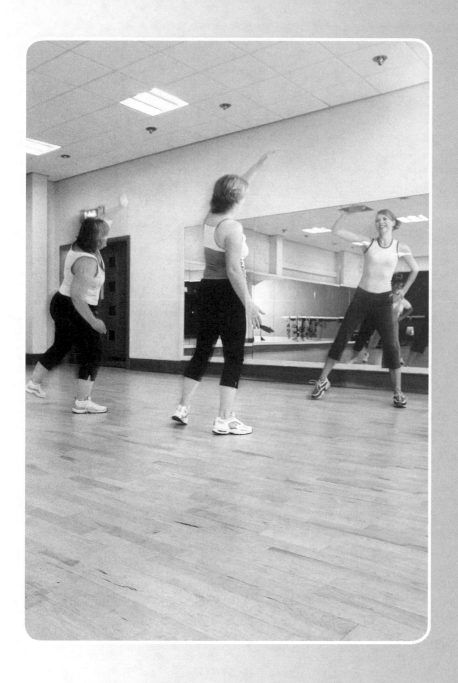

CHAPTER 4

Interventions for Women

Women are typically less likely to participate in regular physical activity or exercise than men (USDHHS, 2005). Compared to active women, those who are sedentary are at significantly higher risk of biological conditions such as heart disease (Duncan, 2006), type 2 diabetes (Jeon, Lokken, Hu, & van Dam, 2007), osteoporosis (Martyn-St. James & Carroll, 2006), and psychological conditions such as depression and anxiety (Kugler, Seelbach, & Kruskemper, 1994).

To counteract this low rate of physical activity and exercise participation in women, researchers and practitioners have begun to design, implement, and evaluate physical activity interventions specifically for women. A mistake that is often made in attempting to increase activity in women is to assume that women's activity and intensity preferences are similar to those of men. Preferences may be similar some of the time, but in many cases, women have very different activity preferences in terms of mode and intensity (Ransdell, Vener, & Sell, 2004; White, Ransdell, Vener, & Flohr, 2005). Specifically, women often prefer to walk or participate in group exercise at a moderate intensity, whereas men prefer to play team sports and work out more vigorously. Given the need to more thoroughly examine ways to encourage women to participate in health-enhancing levels of physical activity, the purpose of this chapter is to (a) summarize factors related to successful physical activity interventions for women, (b) discuss barriers to physical activity in women and strategies for overcoming them, and (c) highlight various aspects of some of the most successful programs to date.

Factors Related to Successful Physical Activity Interventions

Several researchers have reviewed factors that predict participation in and adherence to physical activity in women (Eyler et al., 2002; Lemmon, Ludwig, Howe, Ferguson-Smith, & Barbeau, 2007; Osuji, Lovegreen, Elliott, & Brownson, 2006; Sallis, Hovell, & Hofstetter, 1992; Scharff, Homan, Krueter, & Brennan, 1999; White et al., 2005). We reviewed the literature on this topic and chose to focus on four unique factors related to designing and implementing successful physical activity interventions for women. In addition, intervention specialists are encouraged to consider the basic strategies suggested in the introduction (e.g., establishing a theoretical basis, finding meta-analyses with effect sizes, and using focus groups). Undoubtedly, other factors may affect adherence and participation in women; however, we selected the specific factors that we believe are most modifiable for facilitating change.

The four factors that are related to a successful physical activity intervention for women are as follows:

■ Designing activities that will enhance self-efficacy, activity enjoyment, and social support

- Offering both co-ed and single-sex opportunities for physical activity
- Recommending both moderate and vigorous activities
- Providing opportunities for personal contact with a fitness professional

In the sections that follow, each of these factors is covered in more detail.

Psychological Factors

Several studies have demonstrated the importance of increasing self-efficacy in women to facilitate their participation in and maintenance of physical activity (Brassington, Atienza, Perczek, Dilorenzo, & King, 2002; McAuley, Jerome, Marquez, Elavsky, & Blissmer, 2003; Oman & King, 1998; Wilbur, Miller, Chandler, & McDewitt, 2003). Self-efficacy is defined as situation-specific self-confidence, so in this context, self-efficacy means self-confidence with physical activity abilities.

To increase self-efficacy, activities for previously sedentary women should do the following:

- Emphasize moderate intensity (especially initially, until women get used to being more active).
- Be progressive in nature—both in terms of skill development and intensity level. In other words, the program should start out with activities that are simple and easy to learn so women will experience success, instead of starting out with difficult activities that will "weed out" women who are not used to activity.
- Highlight role models who are from similar backgrounds as the women participating in the program.
- Teach goal-setting techniques because successfully achieving goals builds confidence; participants should focus on *process* goals (i.e., exercising 3 days a week) instead of *product* goals (i.e., losing 10 pounds in 2 weeks).
- Teach about self-monitoring techniques such as logs and pedometers because learning these techniques sensitize women to their current level of activity and inform them about how well they are doing or what they might do to improve.
- Teach about the importance of positive self-talk; many women say negative things to themselves, which can derail their development of self-efficacy.
- Increase activity above the current level—and minimize the focus on achieving instant weight loss or obtaining the perfect body.

Whether a woman *enjoys* a specific type of exercise is another factor that could affect continued participation in activity (Dacey, Baltzell, & Zaichkowsky, 2003; Nies, Vollman, & Cook, 1999). Enjoyment of activity could be affected by exercise or activity intensity (e.g., moderate or vigorous), duration (e.g., multiple short bouts or one long continuous bout), mode (e.g., walking or lifting weights), or social setting (e.g., health club or home). One of the keys to facilitating enjoyment in women is giving them choices as far as activities and exercise intensity. Women should be encouraged to try various types or modes of physical activity until they find something they like to do. If they like what they are doing, they are more likely to continue doing it on a regular basis. Additionally, exercise classes as part of a program should be flexible and offer a variety of alternatives to activities that are difficult. For example, a yoga instructor who offers modifications for women who cannot do certain poses encourages women to continue to participate in the yoga class.

Social support, or the encouragement or assistance a person receives from her family, friends, coworkers, or health professionals, is an important correlate of activity in many women (Eyler et al., 2002; Oka, King, & Young, 1995; Scharff et al., 1999). In one study, women who did vigorous activities such as running or aerobics enjoyed social contact more than women who participated in moderate activities such as yoga or walking. In addition, women who participated in vigorous physical activity felt that being part of a group was integral to their involvement and that having camaraderie with a friend helped them maintain vigorous physical activity (Dacey et al., 2003). Unfortunately, participation in activity may stop or stall when significant others

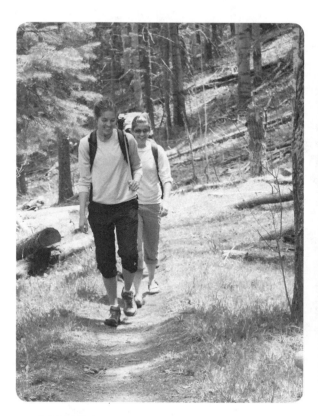
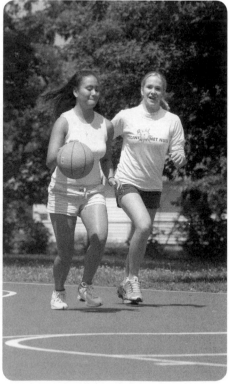

Encouraging women to try various activities so that they find what they like to do will increase the likelihood that they will continue to be physically active.

are not supportive of a physically active lifestyle. Some believe that social support is a more influential factor in the initiation stage of activity, but may not be as much of a factor in the maintenance of long-term physical activity in women (Courneya & McAuley, 1995).

Women-Only Participation Opportunities

Another factor that has been linked to increased participation in physical activity for some women is offering activities in a women-only setting. Although this concept has been developed and tested in school settings (Derry, 2002; McKenzie, Prochaska, Sallis, & LaMaster, 2004) and community settings (Ransdell et al., 2003b, 2004), there is room for additional research designed to discover why and how women-only programming works. Women-only programming works well for women who have body image issues or social physique anxiety (Finkenberg, Dinucci, McCune, Chenette, & McCoy, 1998), women who have been previously sedentary or who have not had extensive instruction in sports or physical activities (Derry, 2002), and women who do not want to participate in activity with men present because of religious beliefs (Benn, 2006).

Derry (2002) interviewed several female students who participated in both co-ed and female-only physical education classes and found that in female-only classes, girls felt more comfort and support from female peers, less fear of failure and embarrassment, more opportunity for self-growth, and improved athletic ability. Female teachers reported less off-task behavior in gender-segregated physical education classes compared to co-ed classes. It is likely that some women prefer a female-only activity environment, but more research is needed in this area.

Physical Activity Intensity

A third factor that has been instrumental in facilitating increases in physical activity in women is the recommendation of moderate to vigorous intensity levels (Anton et al., 2005; Cox, Burke, Gorely, Beilin, & Puddey, 2003; Ekkekakis & Lind, 2006). Women, compared to men, may not want to sweat, shower, or participate in vigorous-intensity activities, including sports. Most women, in fact, prefer walking as their mode of activity—especially during the initial stages of an exercise program (Jakicic, Winters, Lang, & Wing, 1999). It is therefore important to acknowledge these activity preferences and offer programming that will address the activity and intensity preferences of women.

Regular Contact With a Fitness Professional

Providing educational opportunities and personal contact with a fitness professional can dramatically influence the success of a physical activity intervention for women. White and colleagues (2005) reported that women who felt supported by their exercise or fitness instructors were more likely to adhere to a program compared to those who were not able to connect with their instructors. In a follow-up qualitative study, Huberty and colleagues (2008) reported that women who participated in a university-based fitness program and maintained physical activity participation over the long term believed that exercise leadership and connecting with a fitness professional contributed to their self-efficacy and were important determinants of their success. Given the importance of having qualified fitness professionals work within a program, program planners should make sure that those who are hired to lead programs have degrees, credentials, or certifications. Failure to hire qualified fitness professionals to lead programs may result in a higher-than-desirable failure, injury, or dropout rate.

Barriers to Physical Activity and Strategies for Overcoming Them

Knowing the factors related to designing successful physical activity interventions for women is an important way to start planning a future intervention. Identifying barriers and strategies for overcoming these barriers is the next step toward a successful intervention. For example, if a program planner fails to consider that a lack of child care is a major reason women don't participate in physical activity interventions, and doesn't provide child care for participants, the rate of adherence will be lower than usual, and this is one of the easier barriers to accommodate.

Barriers to physical activity are typically divided into three categories: personal, environmental, and social. One major *personal* barrier to physical activity is a lack of time. Women who lack time should be encouraged to try multitasking or riding a stationary bicycle while watching TV or reading. *Environmental* barriers (which are covered in more detail in chapter 8) include the cost of facilities and equipment, crime, traffic patterns, and weather. If weather is inclement or crime is a concern, women should be encouraged to walk together or indoors at a mall. A *social* barrier that presents significant challenges for women is a lack of social support from family or friends. Women who do not feel social support for their activities should try to encourage their family members or friends to join them in activity or explain why participating in exercise is important. Table 4.1 lists more barriers specific to women and strategies for overcoming them. Intervention specialists are encouraged to know as much about these barriers as possible so they can anticipate them and develop strategies for overcoming them (which they can discuss with intervention participants).

In addition to knowing about *general* barriers of women attempting to increase physical activity (table 4.1), it is important to assess *specific* barriers for a given group. Barriers for one group may differ from those for another group. For example, older white women may have different barriers than minority women of child-bearing age. The questionnaire presented in figure 4.1 uses the material covered in table 4.1 to illustrate one way to identify women's barriers to physical activity and brainstorm ways to overcome them. Attention to barriers and strategies for overcoming them should result in increased activity.

TABLE 4.1 **Barriers to Physical Activity in Women and Suggested Strategies for Overcoming Them**

Barrier	Strategies for overcoming barrier
Personal	
Lack of time	Schedule PA into your day or use active commuting
Low self-confidence	Use progressive programming (e.g., gradual increase in intensity or complexity of skill); seek feedback; provide practice opportunities for skill development
High social physique anxiety (i.e., fear of public presentation of the body)	Work out at home or in small groups of similar women
Lack of money for programs	Choose inexpensive activities (walking, using household equipment or stretch bands for resistance training)
Lack of knowledge about PA programs	Take a class on something you've always wanted to learn; work with a fitness professional to learn more about fitness concepts
Fear of injury	Take a class from a qualified professional; start slowly; use proper progressions and equipment
Dislike of sweating and vigorous activity	Use lower-intensity activity and go longer
Failure to gain instant gratification (weight loss)	Talk with professionals about realistic expectations and do it for fun
Procrastination or low motivation	Find a workout partner; exercise with friends; use music during exercise; put workout equipment in a well-lit, motivating place
Illusions of invincibility	Read information about the physical and psychological health benefits of physical activity
Environmental	
Lack of child care	Go to a gym with child care; partner with other families; do family-oriented activities
Expensive facilities and equipment	Choose inexpensive activities (e.g., check out fitness DVDs from the library; walk at the mall, in the neighborhood with a dog, or at a local high school track)
High crime	Work out with a *big* dog or friends
Inflexible work schedule	Work out before or after work; schedule workouts into your day (e.g., three bouts of 10 minutes, walk to a colleague's desk rather than send an e-mail, use the stairs instead of the elevator)
Bad weather	Work out inside (e.g., walk in a mall or use a DVD at home)
Excessive traffic	Find quiet, peaceful places to exercise; work out indoors
No neighborhood connectivity	Work with others to make neighborhoods more connected or work out indoors

(continued) ▷

TABLE 4.1 *(continued)*

Social	
Lack of programming for girls and women	Start a club or activity group in your area
Culturally inappropriate activities	Find activities that are culturally appropriate; work out with others to become more comfortable with activities outside your comfort zone
Prefer other leisure activities such as reading, knitting, watching TV	Listen to books on tape while working out; listen to NPR or another favorite radio show while exercising; knit or watch TV while working out
Lack of social support from friends, spouse, significant other, family	Find activities that your friends and family like to do
Caregiving responsibilities	Develop home-based activities

Potential Barriers

Following is a list of potential barriers women face when they try to participate in physical activity. Please place a check mark next to the barriers that interfere with your ability to participate in physical activity on a regular basis (i.e., at least weekly).

Personal Barriers

_____ Lack of time

_____ Low self-confidence

_____ Procrastination or low motivation

_____ Fear of being ridiculed when exercising in public (i.e., exercise makes me feel self-conscious)

_____ Lack of money

_____ Lack of knowledge about physical activity

_____ Fear of injury

_____ Dislike of sweating or vigorous physical activity

_____ Failure to gain instant gratification (e.g., weight loss)

_____ Exercise is hard work and it makes me tired

_____ Exercise is hard because I am unhealthy/sick/injured

_____ Other:_____

_____ Other:_____

Environmental Barriers

_____ Lack of child care

_____ High crime rate

_____ Inflexible work schedule

_____ Bad weather

_____ Excessive traffic

_____ Neighborhood streets are not connected or pleasant to walk on

_____ Places to exercise are inconvenient

_____ Other:_____

_____ Other:_____

Social Barriers

_____ Lack of programming for girls and women

_____ Prefer other (less active) leisure activities

_____ Lack of social support from spouse or significant other

_____ Lack of social support from family

_____ Lack of social support from friends

_____ Caregiving responsibilities (children, disabled, elderly)

_____ Other:_____

_____ Other:_____

Top Three Barriers

Please list the three most significant challenges to your ability to participate in physical activity on a regular basis.

1. _____

2. _____

3. _____

Solutions for Overcoming the Top Three Barriers

Here you can brainstorm about ways to overcome your barriers. Please fill in your personal solutions to your top three barriers.

1. _____

_____

_____

2. _____

_____

_____

3. _____

_____

_____

FIGURE 4.1 Sample questionnaire for identifying women's barriers to physical activity and brainstorming solutions for overcoming those barriers.

From L. Ransdell, M. Dinger, J. Huberty, and K. Miller, 2009, *Developing Effective Physical Activity Programs* (Champaign, IL: Human Kinetics).

Sample Successful Interventions

In addition to summarizing factors related to successful interventions and barriers to physical activity participation in women, intervention specialists should also examine a number of interventions with women that have successfully increased physical activity behavior. Several programs are highlighted in this section to provide the tools necessary for success in this endeavor.

WISEWOMAN

WISEWOMAN (Well-Integrated Screening and Evaluation for Women Across the Nation) is a multisite, NIH-funded trial designed to remove health-related racial and ethnic disparities by providing screening and interventions for middle-aged uninsured or underinsured women (Will, Farris, Sanders, Stockmyer, & Finkelstein, 2004). The initial goal of the study was to reduce disparities in breast and cervical cancer screening. However, the most recent arm of this study was designed to reduce cardiovascular disease (CVD) risk (Stoddard, Palombo, Troped, Sorensen, & Will, 2004). Participants (n = 1,443; mean age = 58 y; mean BMI = 28.7 kg/m^2) from four states were randomly assigned to either an enhanced intervention (EI) or a minimal intervention (MI).

Both EI and MI sites received CVD risk factor screening; counseling from health professionals; and education, referral, and follow-up. The EI, which was grounded in social cognitive theory and the socioecological model, also received one-on-one nutrition and physical activity programming, access to organized walking groups, and a cultural festival. Baseline and 12-month postintervention data were collected for blood pressure, total cholesterol, number of servings of fruits and vegetables, and level of moderate to vigorous physical activity. Compared to women in the MI group, participants in the EI group reported a significantly larger increase in physical activity (18 vs. 6%), but no other significant changes in health variables (Stoddard et al., 2004).

An entire issue of the *Journal of Women's Health* (volume 13, number 5, 2004) was devoted to describing various arms of the study and related results. Readers are referred to this journal issue for more information on WISEWOMAN. One of the papers in the series described best practices for WISEWOMAN (Farris, Haney, & Dunet, 2004). Table 4.2 is adapted and modified from this paper to show the process of planning, implementing, and evaluating a large-scale intervention.

impACT

Another study that provides a model intervention for underserved women is impACT (Albright et al., 2005). This study was designed to increase physical activity in a multiethnic sample of low-income women (n = 72; 32 ± 10 years), the majority of whom were Latina. Women in the study received 2 months of weekly classes that lasted 1 hour each. During classes, behavior change strategies and motivational readiness for physical activity were addressed. After this initial 2-month period, women were randomly assigned

TABLE 4.2   **WISEWOMAN Success Criteria for Physical Activity and Nutrition (Lifestyle) Interventions**

Planning	Implementing	Evaluating
Develop		
Staff hired **Success indicator:** Expertise in intervention development	Develop intervention protocol **Success indicators:** • Consider theory, evidence, values, and context • Pilot test with staff • Pilot test with participants	Quality intervention developed **Success indicators:** • Theory based • Evidence based • Culturally appropriate • Successful in pilot testing
Implement		
Intervention staff hired and trained **Success indicators:** • Expertise in providing PA interventions • Trained on intervention	Implement intervention **Success indicators:** • Participation rates • Retention • Participant satisfaction • Staff satisfaction	Quality intervention implemented **Success indicator:** Participant knowledge, attitudes, awareness increase or improve
Outcomes		
A well-planned and well-implemented intervention improves behavioral and physiological health outcomes. **Success indicators:** • Behavior change • Risk factor reduction • Morbidity and mortality reduction • Racial disparities reduction		

Adapted, by permission, from R.P Farris, D.M. Haney, and D.O. Dunet, 2004, "Expanding the evidence for health promotion: Developing best practices for WISEWOMAN," *Journal of Women's Health* 13(5): 634-643.

to a 10-month intervention in which they received mailed newsletters only or mailed newsletters plus home-based counseling and additional information and feedback. Women who received the newsletter plus phone counseling and individualized programming expended significantly more energy in physical activity compared to those who received only the newsletter.

SWEAT (Sedentary Women Exercising Adherence Trial)

Cox and colleagues (2003) published research related to the SWEAT (Sedentary Women Exercising Adherence Trial) study. This 18-month study followed 115 initially sedentary women between the ages of 40 and 65 to determine whether an exercise program that begins with 6 months of supervision led to greater retention and adherence to regular activity compared to an unsupervised home-based program. Compared to those in the home-based program, the group that received initial supervision had higher retention and adherence rates to the program, and their energy expenditure was higher.

Moms in Motion

Moms in Motion, developed by Cramp & Brawley (2006), tested the efficacy of a standard exercise treatment compared to a standard exercise treatment plus a mediated cognitive-behavioral intervention. The six mediated counseling sessions focused on things such as self-monitoring of physical activity, goal setting, identifying and overcoming barriers, and relapse prevention. Four weeks of home-based follow-up was provided (e.g., one phone call per week) to attenuate the problem of "letting go" of the program leaders. Results of this program were positive in that compared to women in the standard exercise treatment group, women who received the standard program plus mediated cognitive behavioral intervention reported greater change in moderate physical activity, increased changes in proximal outcome expectancies (e.g., they learned how to make their outcomes of the program more realistic), increased barrier efficacy (e.g., they felt more able to deal with barriers to exercise), and increased cohesion and collaboration.

Project STRIDE

Bess Marcus teamed up with several colleagues to develop Project Stride, a program designed to examine the efficacy of non-face-to-face approaches to increasing physical activity behavior (Marcus et al., 2007). In this study, a group of individuals ($n = 239$; mostly women [82% of sample]) who received phone- or print-based, individualized, motivationally tailored feedback were compared to a contact-control group that received general information about health promotion (so they were still contacted regularly). They also had the option to receive the intervention after serving as the control group for 12 months. At the end of 6 months, participation in moderate physical activity (measured in minutes) was significantly and similarly increased in the print and phone intervention groups, while it remained unchanged in the control group. After 1 year, participants who received print materials maintained a higher level of participation in physical activity compared to those who received the phone intervention or served in the control group. The authors concluded that both phone and print media increased participation in physical activity during the initial 6 months of the program; however, print media may be more important for helping individuals maintain participation in physical activity for longer than 6 months. In addition, it is possible that phone and print-based interventions may be quite effective with women given their household responsibilities related to caregiving, homemaking, and child care.

Another paper from this study described a mediation analysis designed to determine which processes of change from the transtheoretical model were best able to predict changes in physical activity behavior (Napolitano et al.,

2008). Researchers concluded that the impact of the print- and phone-based interventions was mostly due to increases in behavioral processes.

DAMET (Daughters and Mothers Exercising Together) and GET FIT (Generations Exercising Together for Fitness)

In the DAMET and GET FIT studies, daughters and mothers, or daughters, mothers, and grandmothers, participated in physical activity programs that included fitness-building activities, recreational activities, and behavior management principles. These programs used components of the social cognitive theory to increase physical activity behavior in girls and their mothers and grandmothers, and change several psychological variables often associated with adherence to physical activity and overall well-being and self-worth. For more information on these studies, see Ransdell, Oakland, and Taylor (2003a); Ransdell, Robertson, Ornes, and Moyer-Mileur (2004); and Ransdell et al. (2003b).

African American Women Fight Cancer With Fitness (FCF)

Yancy and colleagues (2006) tested the effectiveness of an 8-week culturally sensitive nutrition and physical activity intervention for 366 healthy, obese African American women. Participants were separated into two groups. Both groups were given a free membership to a black-owned health and fitness club. One group received information about developing a balanced exercise regimen (e.g., flexibility, strength, and aerobic activities), and the other group attended sessions on cancer prevention and overall lifestyle improvement. The retention rate in this study was exceptional (71% in both groups). Women in both groups improved their 1-mile (1.6 km) walk-run times; however, after 2 months, women from the exercise regimen group were not as fit as determined by follow-up testing. Women who received the cancer prevention information in addition to the free membership were able to maintain changes in their aerobic fitness over the long term. The authors of this study concluded that giving a free 1-year membership to the black-owned health and fitness club was a more potent motivator than education and social support. Clearly, more research in this area is warranted.

Lifestyle Education for Activity Program (LEAP)

Several top researchers from southern universities planned a study to test the effects of a comprehensive school-based intervention on physical activity among 2,744 diverse high school girls in 14 South Carolina counties (Pate et al., 2005). Half of the schools were assigned to the "typical PE curricula" that was not choice based, focused on skill development, and did not address gender differences in activity preferences. The other half of the schools were assigned to the LEAP program, which was designed to change instructional practices and the school environment to make changes in physical and health education, the school environment, school health services, faculty and staff health promotion practices, and family involvement. Components of the social ecological model were used.

Specifically, the LEAP program was designed to (a) enhance self-efficacy and enjoyment of physical activity, (b) teach physical activity and behavioral skills needed to adopt healthy lifestyles, (c) involve girls in moderate to vigorous physical activity 50% or more of PE class time, (d) include more gender-specific and girl-friendly choice-based instruction, (e) emphasize role modeling of active behaviors, (f) increase communication about and advertising of physical activity, and (g) encourage family and community members to join the effort to increase girls' levels of activity. Results of this study are positive in that the percentage of girls who met the guidelines for increased intensity and duration of activity increased, and the prevalence of regular vigorous physical activity was 8% higher in the LEAP schools compared to control schools. This study is one of the first to show that changes in a school-based curriculum can facilitate an increase in vigorous physical activity in high school girls.

GETTING STARTED

❑ Use low- to moderate-intensity physical activity.

❑ Recommend 10-minute bouts of activity rather than long sessions.

❑ Use activities that enhance self-efficacy (e.g., proper progressions, role models, goal setting, self-monitoring, and positive self-talk).

❑ Enhance enjoyment by building in opportunities for success; manipulating exercise intensity, duration, or type; and providing recommendations for modifications of activities.

❑ Facilitate social support from family, friends, and exercise instructors.

❑ Offer co-ed and women-only programming.

❑ Provide opportunities for personal contact with a fitness professional.

Summary

The fact that women are commonly less active than men is a public health problem that needs immediate attention. Compared to men, women prefer different types and intensities of activity, and different factors relate to their participation. Therefore, it is important that physical activity intervention specialists consider employing strategies to affect not only physical well-being, but also the psychological factors that predict activity in women (e.g., self-efficacy, enjoyment, and social support). Program planners should also consider offering women-only participation opportunities, modifying physical activity intensity, facilitating regular contact with fitness professionals, using focus groups to ascertain activity preferences, and learning about barriers to activity in this population. Contrary to several years ago when interventions were not gender specific, a variety of successful gender-specific programs are available as models for future program planning.

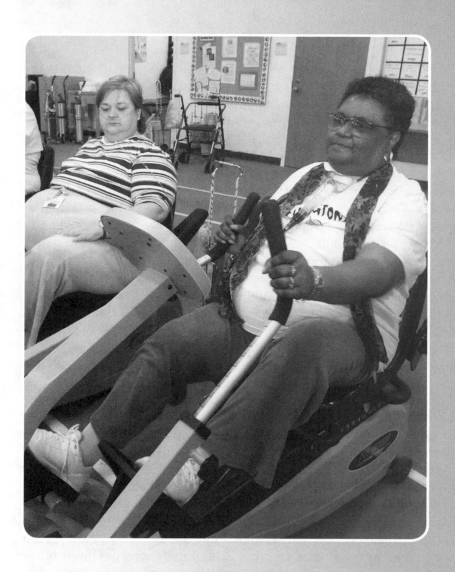

CHAPTER 5

Interventions for Obese and Overweight People

Excess body fat, also known as overweight or obesity, is a health problem that has increased dramatically during the last few decades (National Center for Health Statistics [NCHS] Health E-Stats, 2008). Compared to normal-weight people, obese and overweight people have higher risk of type 2 diabetes, hypertension, coronary heart disease, stroke, pulmonary alterations (e.g., sleep apnea), orthopedic problems, cancer, and premature mortality (Calle & Kaaks, 2004; Colditz, Willett, Rotnitzky, & Manson, 1995; Huang et al., 1998; Manson et al., 2007; Rexrode et al., 1997; Willett et al., 1995).

Obesity and overweight conditions also have psychological and social consequences. Overweight children are sometimes excluded from activities in which normal-weight children participate, and they are often viewed negatively by their peers. In addition, overweight and obese children and adults have reported lower self-esteem, increased depression, and other negative psychological conditions that affect their social interactions, relationships, and performance in school and work (Baum & Forehand, 1984; Carey, Hegvik, & McDevitt, 1988; Mathus-Vliegen, 2007; Puhl & Brownell, 2006). Physical and psychological health problems related to this explosion of overweight and obesity have prompted some researchers to predict that this generation will be the first that will not live longer than their parents (Olshansky et al., 2005).

Given the physical and psychological health risks of obesity, it is important for physical activity specialists to approach programs for these people somewhat differently than they would programs for their normal-weight counterparts. For example, overweight or obese people may feel more fatigued after participating in activity, or they may have more intense physiological and psychological reactions to exercise (Ekkekakis & Lind, 2006). When compared to normal-weight people, overweight and obese people exercise at a higher percentage of their peak oxygen uptake ($\dot{V}O_2$peak), and at a higher percentage of their maximum heart rate. They also report higher ratings of perceived exertion at the same workload (Ekkekakis & Lind, 2006). This may affect their motivation to start and continue exercise. Additionally, overweight or obese people may negatively appraise themselves while exercising or experience high levels of anxiety or fear in public exercise settings (Ekkekakis & Lind, 2006). Finally, genetic issues may alter the ability of overweight or obese people to lose weight; therefore, they may quit programs prematurely if they don't see immediate results (i.e., weight loss). Clearly, obesity and overweight are difficult conditions to manage using only physical activity interventions; other lifestyle changes such as dietary intake and stress management should be considered to ensure maximal success.

Two measurements are commonly used to assess whether someone is overweight or obese or to determine whether weight loss is occurring. Body mass index (BMI or kg/m^2) is determined by dividing weight in kilograms by height in meters squared. This technique, although not as accurate for those who are muscular or have above-average bone density, is effective for assessing overweight and obesity prevalence in large populations (e.g., a proportion of citizens in the state of Idaho). Percent body fat, which indicates the percentage of a person's body that consists of fat, is typically assessed using skinfold calipers or hydrostatic weighing (among other techniques). Percent body fat is a better measure of health status, but measurements must be completed by trained technicians, and it is much more difficult to estimate percent body fat in large samples of people because of the time and cost associated with the process.

When using BMI to categorize adults based on their body weight relative to height, values between 25 and 29.9 kg/m² are considered overweight; adults are considered obese if their BMI is 30 or more kg/m² (National Heart, Lung, and Blood Institute, 1998). Children and adolescents are categorized as "overweight" and "at risk for overweight" rather than "obese" to avoid the negative societal connotations associated with obesity. Using a chart of age- and gender-specific norms, as developed by the working group on childhood obesity from the International Obesity Task Force, children and adolescents are considered overweight if their BMI (kg/m²) is ≥ the 95th percentile; they are considered "at risk for overweight" if their BMI is between the 85th and 95th percentile (Kaur, Hyder, & Poston, 2003). For more information on classifying children and adolescents as overweight or obese, see Bellizzi and Dietz (1999) or Kuczmarski and colleagues (2000).

Women are considered obese if their percent body fat is 30% or higher, and men are considered obese if their percent body fat is 25% or higher, although this can vary with age. It is sometimes more acceptable for older people to have higher percent body fat compared to their younger counterparts (American College of Sports Medicine, 2006).

Worldwide, it is estimated that 1 to 1.7 billion adults are overweight; as many as 300 million adults have been clinically diagnosed with obesity (Deitel, 2003; World Health Organization [WHO], 2008). Americans are contributing to this obesity epidemic (Nothwehr, Snetselaar, & Wu, 2006) in that 65.7% of U.S. adults (20 years old or older) are overweight or obese. Interestingly, urban Samoa has a higher rate of obesity than the United States (i.e., over 75% of the population is obese), and some urban areas of China, a country of people thought to be relatively lean, have a prevalence of obesity as high as 20% (WHO, 2008). In Europe, obesity in men over 50 years of age ranges from 12.8% (in Sweden) to 20.2% (in Spain), and obesity in women from the same age group ranges from 12.3% (in Switzerland) to 25.6% (in Spain) (Andreyeva, Michaud, & van Soest, 2007). Interestingly, experts from the WHO have suggested that Asians may be more vulnerable to weight-related diseases; for that reason, the optimal BMI recommended for that population is 18.5 to 23 kg/m² (lower than the BMI of 25 kg/m² used to classify Americans and Europeans as overweight; Deitel, 2003).

In the United States and around the world, the prevalence of overweight and obesity has increased steadily over the years in both men and women, and among all ages, racial and ethnic groups, and educational levels (Andreyeva, Michaud, & van Soest, 2007; Janssen et al., 2005; Weight Control Information Network, 2007). From 1960 to 2002, the prevalence of overweight increased from 44.8 to 65.7% in U.S. adults; the prevalence of obesity during this same time period more than doubled among adults from 13.3 to 30.5%, with most of this rise occurring in the past 20 years (Weight Control Information Network, 2007; see figure 5.1). Minorities and those with lower socioeconomic status, especially of African American and Mexican American descent, face a higher risk of obesity than their white counterparts (Fiore, Travis, Whalen, Auinger, & Ryan, 2006; Hedley et al., 2004).

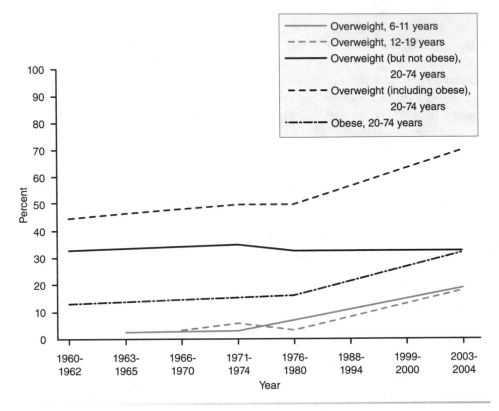

FIGURE 5.1 The prevalence of overweight and obesity in American adults (1960-2002).

Reprinted from Center for Disease Control and Prevention, National Center for Health Statistics, Health, United States, 2006, Data from the National Health and Nutrition Examination Survey.

As obesity rates have continued to rise, so have associated medical costs. Direct medical costs include preventive, diagnostic, and treatment costs associated with obesity; indirect costs are those associated with decreased productivity, absenteeism, sickness, premature death, and other conditions that are an indirect result of overweight or obesity (Centers for Disease Control and Prevention, 2007). Direct and indirect medical costs associated with obesity in the United States were as high as $92.6 billion per year in 2002 (Centers for Disease Control and Prevention, 2007).

Given the obesity crisis, the health consequences of overweight and obesity, and the need to encourage overweight and obese people to participate in health-enhancing levels of physical activity, the purpose of this chapter is to (a) summarize factors related to successful physical activity interventions for overweight and obese people, (b) discuss barriers to physical activity and strategies for overcoming them, and (c) highlight various aspects of some of the most successful programs to date.

Factors Related to Successful Physical Activity Interventions

When delineating the factors most related to successful physical activity interventions for those who are obese or overweight, several important sources were considered: recent meta-analyses on various aspects of weight loss (Anderson, Konz, Frederich, & Wood, 2001; Garrow & Summerbell, 1995; Miller, Koceja, & Hamilton, 1997; Snethen, Broome, & Cashin, 2006), systematic reviews on weight loss (Curioni & Lourenco, 2005; Jakicic & Otto, 2006; Kaur et al., 2003; Shaw, O'Rourke, Del Mar, and Kenardy, 2005), and information from the National Weight Control Registry, a database that contains information from over 5,000 people who lost a significant amount of weight (at least 30 lb, or 13.6 kg) and have been able to keep the weight off for an extended period of time (National Weight Control Registry, 2007). This combination of resources leads us to recommend the following five factors when designing a physical activity intervention for those who are overweight or obese:

- Combine diet and exercise lifestyle changes with behavioral and cognitive strategies for the most favorable short- and long-term results.
- Encourage participation in high levels of physical activity to maintain weight loss.
- Recommend that participants select the intensity of their activities so they will experience success and have fun.
- Involve participants' family members, peers, and significant others in the lifestyle change process.
- Shift the focus away from weight loss and toward other benefits such as increasing physical activity, improving health, and relieving stress.

Combining Diet and Exercise for Improvements

In a meta-analysis, Miller and colleagues (1997) examined 25 years of data from 493 subjects to determine the impact of short-term interventions (mean = 15 weeks) on weight loss. The participants in this study were mostly women, about 40 years old, with a BMI of 33.4 kg/m^2. Results were compared based on programs that used diet only, exercise only, or diet plus exercise interventions. Participants in the diet plus exercise groups lost the most weight (24 lb, or 10.9 kg) over the typical 15-week period, whereas participants in the diet only group lost an average of 23 pounds (10.4 kg), and those who participated only in exercise without additional dietary manipulation lost only 6.4 pounds (2.9 kg). The key findings in this study are that (a) the group that changed both diet and exercise habits lost the most weight and they were able to keep the weight off for a longer period of time after completing the intervention, and (b) those who exercise only, and do not manipulate their diets, should not expect significant weight loss.

Several researchers have concluded that targeting changes in both diet and exercise habits can facilitate greater *loss* of fat weight and *preservation* of calorie-burning lean body mass, compared to diet or exercise interventions alone (Anderson, Konz, Frederich, & Wood, 2001; Curioni & Lourenco, 2005; Garrow & Summerbell, 1995; Miller et al., 1997). In addition, some researchers suggest that the addition of exercise to a weight loss program (versus dieting alone) helps to preferentially reduce unhealthy abdominal fat. Because the majority of health problems related to obesity are linked to abdominal fat, which is deposited near many vital organs, combining diet and exercise in a comprehensive weight loss plan should attenuate the risk of some health problems (You et al., 2006).

Using meta-analytic techniques, Shaw, O'Rourke, Del Mar, and Kenardy (2005) examined the effects of psychological interventions on weight loss. They concluded that compared to simply recommending changes in diet and exercise, adding behavioral and cognitive strategies such as goal setting, positive self-talk, and keeping nutrition and physical activity logs (i.e., self-monitoring) resulted in significantly greater weight reductions. For children and adolescents, strategies such as stimulus control (e.g., substituting sedentary activities with more active ones or storing nonnutritive food out of sight), positive reinforcement for active behaviors, and contracting or reward charts are also effective (Kaur et al., 2003; Snethen et al., 2006).

Contracting consists of writing down SMART goals (specific, measurable, achievable, realistic, and time sensitive) and specifying rewards for reaching them or consequences for failing to reach them. Reward charts emphasize process-oriented goals such as participating in 40 minutes of activity at least 5 days per week. For example, each time a person completes a goal, he or she receives a star or sticker on a calendar. Figure 5.2 contains a sample of a SMART goal chart that can be used with people participating in a physical activity program.

Encouraging Participation in High Levels of PA

Weight loss is not fast or simple. The fact that it requires a significant, whole-hearted, personal investment in a lifestyle change can deter some people from trying. The mantra spoken by professionals in our field is that 3,500 calories equal a pound of fat. Therefore, to lose a pound, one should cut calories from dietary intake and increase caloric expenditure above what is "typical." For example, if a person walks 3 miles (4.5 km), 5 days a week and expends 1,500 additional calories per week and eliminates 200 calories of desserts 5 days a

Process Goals

In the space below, write three *process,* or short-term, goals related to your regular participation in physical activity. These goals should target a time period no longer than a week. An example of a process goal is: "I want to participate in 40 minutes of walking at least 4 days this week" or "I want to go to yoga class twice this week."

1. _____

_____

_____

_____

S   M   A   R   T

2. _____

_____

_____

_____

S   M   A   R   T

3. _____

_____

_____

_____

S   M   A   R   T

Product Goals

In the space below, write three *product,* or long-term, goals related to what you expect to happen as a result of your participation in physical activity for a month or more. An example of a product, or outcome, goal is: "I want to walk my 2-mile route faster in 4 weeks than I did this week" or "I want to lose 4 pounds in a month."

1. _____

_____

_____

_____

S   M   A   R   T

2. _____

_____

_____

_____

S   M   A   R   T

FIGURE 5.2   SMART Goal Chart for participants in a physical activity program.

From L. Ransdell, M. Dinger, J. Huberty, and K. Miller, 2009, *Developing Effective Physical Activity Programs* (Champaign, IL: Human Kinetics).

3. _____

_____

_____

_____

S   M   A   R   T

Go back through your goals above and make sure they are SMART goals. Ask yourself the following questions for each goal and circle the letter that corresponds with each question if the goal meets the letter:

Is it (S)pecific enough?

Is it (M)easurable (so I can tell when I have reached my goal)?

Is it (A)chievable based on the amount of time and effort I am committing?

Is it (R)ealistic based on my past accomplishments (and the accomplishments of others in a similar situation)?

Is it (T)ime sensitive (in other words, does it have a deadline?)

Reward for Goal Accomplishment

In the space below, identify any rewards you will allow yourself if you meet one to three of your goals.

_____

_____

_____

_____

_____

_____

FIGURE 5.2 *(continued)*

week (1,000 calories), this results in a deficit of 2,500 calories per week. With these adjustments to caloric expenditure and caloric intake, it would take that person approximately 2 weeks to lose 1.5 pounds (0.7 kg). Most people want to lose weight more quickly than that, however. One way to increase the caloric expenditure of exercise is to exercise longer or more intensely— which is not always possible for someone who is overweight or obese. Longer or more intense exercise results in a larger number of calories burned, and it facilitates continued calorie burning even after the exercise has stopped (this phenomenon is known as postexercise oxygen consumption). Another option for increasing energy expenditure is to substitute participation in sedentary activities such as watching television or playing computer or video games with more active pursuits such as riding a bicycle while watching TV (Fowler-Brown & Kahwati, 2004).

A third option for increasing caloric expenditure is to walk, in-line skate, or bicycle to school or work. This is known as active commuting. Encouraging overweight and obese clients to actively commute to work or school, even over a distance of 2 miles (3.2 km) round trip, can result in an increase in caloric expenditure of 200 calories per day. The following sidebar and table 5.1 contain some additional ideas about how many calories are burned in an exercise session. Readers should note that the higher the intensity of activity, the shorter the activity bout required to burn *similar* numbers of calories compared to a longer, less intense activity bout.

Anderson and colleagues (2001) conducted a meta-analysis with 29 studies to examine the long-term weight loss maintenance of people completing a structured weight loss program. They concluded that those who exercised the most were more able to maintain their weight loss compared to those who exercised less. This ability to maintain weight loss as a result of exercise is a result of an increase in lean body (muscle) mass, an increase in basal metabolic rate (the number of calories burned while resting, which increases with more muscle mass), and the additional calories burned with an exercise bout.

TABLE 5.1   **Selected Activities and Caloric Expenditures for Hypothetical Overweight Men (250 lb/113 kg) and Women (160 lb/72.6 kg) Exercising From 15 to 60 Minutes**

Activity	Calories burned in 15 minutes	Calories burned in 30 minutes	Calories burned in 45 minutes	Calories burned in 60 minutes
Aerobics (moderate) (.065 cal/lb/min)	Men = 244 Women = 156	Men = 488 Women = 312	Men = 731 Women = 468	Men = 975 Women = 624
Basketball (moderate) (.046 cal/lb/min)	Men = 173 Women = 110	Men = 345 Women = 221	Men = 518 Women = 331	Men = 690 Women = 442
Cycling (10 mph) or strength training (.050 cal/lb/min)	Men = 188 Women = 120	Men = 375 Women = 240	Men = 563 Women = 360	Men = 750 Women = 480
Running (11-min mile) or exercising on stair climber or stationary bicycle (vigorous level) (.070 cal/lb/min)	Men = 263 Women = 168	Men = 525 Women = 336	Men = 788 Women = 504	Men = 1,050 Women = 672
Tennis (moderate level) or walking (4.5 mph) (.045 cal/lb/min)	Men = 169 Women = 108	Men = 338 Women = 216	Men = 506 Women = 324	Men = 675 Women = 432

Note: Men typically burn more calories than women because they weigh more, and it "costs" more calories to move more weight. To calculate calories burned for a person who weighs more or less, multiply the energy expenditure factor in the table (e.g., .045 for walking 4.5 mph) times body weight (in pounds) times the length of time of the workout (in minutes).

Based on W.K. Hoeger and S.A. Hoeger, 2009, *Lifetime physical fitness and wellness*, 10th ed. (Belmont, CA: Cengage Learning), 151.

Estimated Amount of Walking and Jogging Needed to Expend 3,500 Calories (and Lose 1 Pound, or 0.45 Kilograms, of Fat)

- Take 40 walks of 15 minutes each
- Take 20 walks of 30 minutes each
- Take 13 walks of 45 minutes each
- Take 10 walks of 60 minutes each
- Jog (11-minute miles) or exercise on a stair climber 26 times for 15 minutes
- Jog or exercise on a stair climber 13 times for 30 minutes
- Jog or exercise on a stair climber 9 times for 45 minutes
- Jog or exercise on a stair climber 6 times for 60 minutes

Based on B.E. Ainsworth et al., 1993, "Compendium of physical activities: Classification of energy costs of human physical activities," *Medicine and Science in Sports and Exercise* 25(1): 71-80.

Recommending Self-Selecting the Intensity of Activities

In studies that examined the effects of exercise intensity on mood, researchers concluded that higher-intensity exercise was associated with undesirable changes in mood and affect (Berger, Motl, Martin, Wilkinson, & Owen, 1999; Parfitt, Rose, & Burgess, 2006). Ekkekakis and Lind (2006) examined whether allowing overweight people on a weight loss regimen to self-select their exercise intensity might increase adherence and therefore improve results. They believed that a self-selected exercise pace would result in more positive self-appraisals, better ratings of pleasure and comfort during exercise, and fewer musculoskeletal problems. They also believed that the lack of autonomy, which is common in group exercise classes (i.e., non-self-selected pace), might limit intrinsic motivation for future exercise participation. Results indicated that women who self-selected their exercise intensity had more positive ratings of perceived exertion, and women who did not self-select their exercise intensity expressed increasing displeasure with the imposed speed over time.

Parfitt and colleagues (2006) indicated that when overweight or obese people self-selected their exercise intensity, they chose an intensity that was high enough to elicit health benefits. Also, study participants reported increased perceived exertion and negative affect during the final stages of a 20-minute exercise bout, providing evidence that multiple shorter (e.g., 10-minute) bouts of activity may promote adherence better than prescribing one longer dose of activity in clients who are overweight or obese.

An additional factor to consider is that humans are hedonistic. Therefore, they pursue activities in which they have fun and feel self-confident. When people are not confident about their abilities, they do not have fun and they tend to avoid participating in these activities. Given that participation in activity is often difficult for those who are overweight or obese, it is important for exercise leaders to include activities that will boost their self-confidence (Palmeira et al., 2007). An exercise leader who wants to boost the self-confidence of a client who is overweight or obese can develop a collaborative plan for self-care that includes an assessment of beliefs, barriers, and supports relative to exercise; design a personal action plan that includes goals beyond simple weight loss; and make sure that a follow-up plan monitors progress (Ash et al., 2006). Additionally, activities should be progressive and appropriate for the client's fitness level.

Involving Others in the Process

Involving family members, peers, and significant others in the process of increased physical activity, lifestyle changes, and weight loss seems to facilitate attaining goals (Caballero, 2004; Neumark-Sztainer, 2005). Neumark-Sztainer (2005) suggested that the two factors that most strongly contribute to a negative weight control environment or unhealthful weight control behaviors are family meal structure and family weight concerns. Specifically, girls who lived in households with unstructured family meals (i.e., they did not eat together often) and excessive concerns about weight were more likely to use unhealthful weight control behaviors compared to their counterparts who did not have excessive concerns about weight and who ate structured family meals. Relative to physical activity, studies have demonstrated that family participation in physical activity can increase aptitude for activity, particularly in people who are overweight and not morbidly obese (Neumark-Sztainer, Kaufmann, & Berry, 1995).

Fiore, Travis, Whalen, Auinger, and Ryan (2006) examined protective factors that prevent obesity in families with parents who are overweight and of normal weight. They found that children with two overweight or obese parents were more likely to be overweight or obese, and that hours per day of television watching and exercise participation were positively and negatively related to BMI, respectively. Interestingly, in this study, compared to their overweight counterparts, adolescents with a healthy weight reported a higher mean head of household educational level, consumed more dietary fiber, and had higher math and reading scores. These findings have implications for the familial factors related to being overweight. Household education, time spent in sedentary (e.g., watching TV) and active pursuits, and fiber consumption seem to play a role in obesity prevention.

Shifting Participant Focus Away From Weight Loss

The prospect of weight loss, at least initially, facilitates extrinsic motivation. Because weight loss is one of the last benefits seen with an exercise program (after psychological changes and other areas of health-related fitness), it is important for exercise professionals to emphasize the more intrinsic benefits of exercise (e.g., increased sense of well-being and goal accomplishment, enhanced self-esteem, stress management, and improved health) (Gillison,

Standage, & Skevington, 2006; Miller et al., 1997; Thomas, 2006). Several researchers have concluded that emphasizing the health benefits of exercise (e.g., feeling more energetic, stress management) rather than weight loss expectations results in more positive outcomes (Neumark-Sztainer, Kaufman, & Berry, 1995; Seger, Spruijt-Metz, & Nolen-Hoeksema, 2006). Helping overweight and obese people shift their motivation from extrinsic to intrinsic involves three basic strategies: (a) promoting activities that facilitate feelings of competence, (b) giving participants control (autonomy) over their program, and (c) encouraging participants to make connections with others (e.g., increase feelings of relatedness or belonging) (Parfitt et al., 2006).

Those with unrealistic weight loss expectations or body shape motives for exercising may develop false hopes and eventually feelings of defeat. If professionals working with overweight or obese clients emphasize intrinsic motives for participating in activity rather than extrinsic motives, this typically results in lower social physique anxiety (i.e., fear of public presentation), depression, and anxiety and higher self-esteem and self-efficacy (Seger et al., 2006).

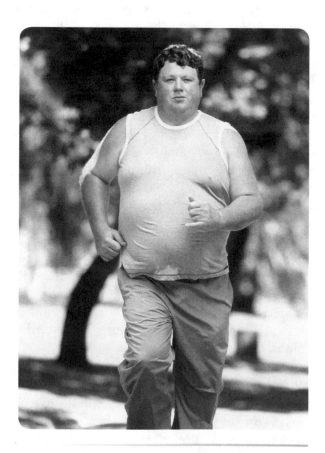

Exercise professionals should emphasize the intrinsic benefits of exercise to prevent the participants from focusing too much on weight loss.

Barriers to Physical Activity and Strategies for Overcoming Them

Overweight and obese people face unique personal, environmental, and social barriers to physical activity participation. Personal barriers include the following:

- The fact that weight loss takes significant time and effort—and many people do not continue to work out when weight loss does not occur quickly
- Low self-confidence because exercise is more difficult and probably less comfortable for overweight and obese people
- Fear of injuries as a result of balance and coordination issues related to carrying around extra weight

To overcome some of these personal barriers, leaders of exercise programs need to develop proper progressions, give positive and corrective feedback, and help participants get to know one another.

In addition to personal barriers, environmental and social barriers exist for this population. One major environmental barrier to activity is that exercise and fitness classes are often designed for those who are already fit. To overcome that barrier, overweight or obese clients should seek workout tapes or CDs that allow them to exercise at their own convenience and comfort level at home. Another option is to seek classes that address their needs specifically (i.e., with modifications for difficult exercises). Table 5.2 presents a detailed summary of barriers and recommended solutions for working with overweight or obese people. As is true with other populations discussed in this book, it is important that those interested in helping overweight and obese people increase their level of physical activity understand these barriers so they can develop strategies for overcoming them.

Sample Successful Interventions

This section describes the characteristics of programs for overweight and obese people. The programs included in this section are unique, innovative, and successful from the standpoint of improving both psychological (e.g., self-esteem, self-efficacy) and physiological (e.g., weight loss, high blood pressure) health.

ALIFE@Work

The primary purpose of the ALIFE@Work study was to evaluate the effectiveness of a lifestyle intervention, delivered by phone or the Internet, on body weight, physical activity, and eating habits in a sample of working men and women; secondary objectives were to compare the effectiveness of phone

TABLE 5.2   Barriers to Physical Activity in Overweight or Obese People and Suggested Strategies for Overcoming Them

Barrier	Strategies for overcoming barrier
Personal	
Significant physical exertion required	Participate in low- to moderate-intensity exercise or self-select the intensity of exercise, or participate in multiple shorter (10-minute) bouts of activity
Low self-confidence	Develop proper progressions; seek feedback from instructor; choose enjoyable activities
Fear of injuries	Take a class from a qualified professional; start slowly; use proper progressions and equipment
Failure to connect with instructor or others in group exercise class	Make efforts to get to know instructor and others in the class; explain your strengths and weaknesses and ask for suggestions
Failure to achieve significant and quick weight loss	Talk with professionals about realistic expectations and ways to increase intrinsic motivation; think about areas other than weight loss that you would like to improve (e.g., muscular strength, aerobic fitness)
Environmental	
Exercise machines that do not accommodate larger body sizes	Exercise at home with customized equipment or tapes or CDs that address the needs of overweight or obese clients
Exercise classes that do not account for differences in baseline fitness or do not provide alternative activities for overweight or obese clients	Learn (or ask) about alternative activities for overweight or obese people; ask for prescreening of health-related fitness prior to activity; develop individualized programs; use tapes or CDs to build fitness and increase confidence in a class setting
Social	
Lack of active overweight or obese role models	Look for classes designed specifically for overweight or obese participants (or classes with participants of a variety of shapes and sizes); find classes taught by overweight or average size instructors
Fear of exercising in public	Exercise at home or in facilities that cater to overweight people
Lack of programming for overweight or obese people	Start a club or activity group in your area
Prefer more sedentary activities such as reading, watching TV, video games, Internet surfing	Figure out a way to multitask while exercising (e.g., listen to books on tape or watch movies while exercising, reward yourself with sedentary activities after you finish exercising)

versus Internet interventions, and to evaluate the cost-effectiveness of the program (van Wier et al., 2006). Participants ($n = 1,386$) were randomly assigned to one of three groups: phone intervention, Internet intervention, and control. Those in the intervention conditions receive 10 lessons spread throughout a

6-month period. Activities were grounded in social cognitive theory. Factors emphasized in the program were (a) identifying behaviors in need of change, (b) setting goals, (c) monitoring progress, (d) modifying environmental cues, and (e) modifying consequences to motivate change. Between sessions, counselors provided feedback to participants either by phone or over the Internet. Results of the study are forthcoming, but this study is important because it is one of the largest obesity prevention programs in recent years.

The Connectors

The Connectors are a group of women who initially decided to lose weight by training for a marathon (Othersen-Gorman, 1999). Inspired by Oprah, this group of approximately 50 women, aged 25 to 56 years old (most of whom are at least 30 lb, or 13.6 kg, overweight) regularly connects online. They chat with each other about the trials and tribulations of training, and they motivate each other to continue. They log on before and after running to discuss running goals, losing weight, and life. This program is a wonderful example of the power of social connections, role modeling, setting goals, and a burning desire to accomplish a physical feat never before thought possible. More information about this program is available at www.nomoreexcuses. net.

Club Ped

The American Diabetes Association sponsors a program called Club Ped (www.diabetes.org/weightloss-and-exercise.jsp). This program, designed specifically for people with diabetes, is a walking club designed to encourage participants to increase their level of physical activity, log on to the Web site and track their steps, compete for prizes when they accomplish goals, and work to minimize the negative impact of diabetes. This program encourages weight loss to lessen the negative impact of the disease, but it also highlights the positive health benefits that can be accomplished with increased physical activity and weight loss.

Energy Up

Energy Up is a 9-month obesity prevention program designed for predominantly minority, inner-city teen girls ($n = 46$) (Chehab, Pfeffer, Vargas, Chen, & Irigoyen, 2007). This program is unique in that it focuses on addictive food avoidance, exercise, and self-esteem building. Girls in this study were made aware that overeating is caused by food addictions that can be prompted by negative self-views and behaviors and triggered by "addictive foods" such as sugar and salt. They are also taught that kind behavior to others and positive affirmations will improve self-esteem. Knowledge about trigger foods, positive self-views, and regular exercise participation helped to facilitate weight loss ranging from 2.9 to 12.9 pounds (1.3 to 5.9 kg). Those who attended more of the sessions reported greater weight loss.

National Weight Control Registry (NWCR)

The NWCR, a database of over 5,000 self-selected people who lost at least 30 pounds (13.6 kg) and have kept it off for at least 1 year, provides significant information about what works relative to weight loss (Klem, Wing, McGuire, Seagle, & Hill, 1997). First, the majority of these people (77%) experienced a "triggering event" (e.g., medical, emotional, or lifestyle) that prompted them to lose weight. Some important dietary manipulations related to maintaining weight loss include limiting fat intake, limiting food quantity, counting calories, and using liquid meal replacements when worried about food intake. The majority (92%) of the people in the database exercised at home, and approximately 33% exercised regularly in groups or with friends. Many areas of their lives improved as a result of weight loss, including quality of life, energy level, physical mobility, mood, self-confidence, and physical health. Approximately half of the participants reported improvements in social interactions, job performance, and the pursuit of hobbies with weight loss.

Multiple or Combined Theory Intervention

Palmeira and colleagues (2007) tested four contemporary theories of health behavior change (e.g., social cognitive theory, transtheoretical model, theory of reasoned action, and the health belief model) in terms of effectiveness in predicting weight loss in a sample of almost 150 middle-aged women. In this study, participants in the intervention group attended 15 weekly meetings lasting 2 hours each. Topics included caloric expenditure of physical activities, apparel for exercise, using pedometers, emotional eating, and preventing lapses. Participants were given an individualized diet and exercise plan designed to induce a caloric deficit of 300 to 500 calories per day. The overall goals of the program were to increase autonomy, social support, and self-efficacy and change social norms to include physical activity. With this type of intervention, the exercise variables that changed the most were barriers, social support, intention to exercise, exercise interest and enjoyment, perceived competence, and intrinsic motivation for exercise. Weight changes in program participants were most associated with changes in self-efficacy, attitudes, and perceived behavioral control.

Polar Weight Management Program (PWMP)

The Polar Weight Management Program (PWMP) is unique in that researchers randomly assigned 74 people into a 32-week personalized fitness program using a heart rate monitor or a standard care program (SCP) (Byrne et al., 2006). Participants in the SCP received a single consultation with advice about increasing physical activity and decreasing energy intake. The goal of this group was to lose no more than 1 kilogram per week. Those in the PWMP group received the standard care session described above, plus, they were given a heart rate monitor and weight management resources that included recommendations for daily energy intake and energy expenditure (based on weight, height, age, sex, target weight, occupational activity, and self-selected exercise intensity). The PWMP program required weekly updates and adjustments according to progress reports. Communication with the researchers was recommended via e-mail. At the completion of the study, those who completed the PWMP lost 3 more kilograms of body weight, 3 more kilograms of fat mass, and 3 more centimeters of waist circumference compared to their counterparts in the SCP.

❏ Encourage people to self-select exercise intensity.

❏ Recommend several 10-minute bouts of physical activity rather than longer sessions—especially for those just getting started.

❏ Require physician permission prior to participation in a program because of the greater health risks and liability associated with physical activity participation in this population.

❏ Realize that overweight and obese people have psychological and physiological issues relative to exercise that differ from those who are of normal weight (e.g., faster fatigue, higher perceived exertion at the same workload, higher level of anxiety about exercising in public, lower self-esteem and self-efficacy related to exercise).

❏ Don't judge the success of a program on weight loss alone; emphasize short-term goals such as participation in physical activity as well as long-term goals related to health and weight loss.

❏ Combine diet and exercise changes with behavioral and cognitive strategies for best results; exercise without dietary changes does not typically result in significant weight loss.

❏ Emphasize that those who lose weight and keep it off participate in high levels of physical activity (e.g., up to 60 minutes of moderate activity daily).

❏ Involve family members and significant others in the lifestyle change process.

❏ Help overweight and obese people make social connections within a class to keep them coming back.

❏ Encourage the use of tapes and CDs at home to develop a baseline fitness level prior to joining a class.

GETTING STARTED

Summary

Exercise and physical activity typically increase feelings of satisfaction and self-confidence, improve physical and psychological health, and enable those who lose weight to maintain that weight loss; however, it is not a magic pill that will transform one's body overnight. The bottom line is that successful weight loss demands attention to multiple competing factors. In today's world in which people want overnight success, the prospect of sticking with a demanding weight loss program is difficult. This chapter provides some concrete strategies for designing an effective program for overweight or obese people, and it recommends some novel and effective model programs from which strategies and tactics can be developed.

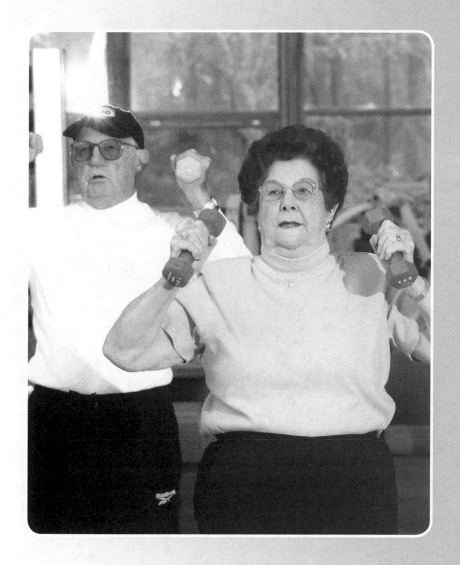

CHAPTER 6

Interventions for Older Adults

Terry-Ann Gibson, PhD

Adults 65 years of age and older are one of the fastest-growing population segments in the United States (U.S. Census Bureau, 2004). Despite the well-documented benefit of physical activity to preserve physical function and health and reduce the severity of chronic diseases, only 8.1% of adults 65 to 74 years of age engage in 10 minutes or more of vigorous physical activity three or four times per week (National Center for Health Statistics, 2004). It is also estimated that 77% of Americans over the age of 65 do not engage in any physical activity (U.S. Department of Health and Human Services, 2005). Part of this may be related to older adults' mistaken belief that physical activity is not safe for them.

The majority of older adults, even those with medical conditions and chronic diseases, can safely participate in physical activities with a few precautions. Preactivity screening can help identify older adults who have increased health risks and possible exercise contraindications. Two self-administered assessments are available: the Physical Activity Readiness Questionnaire or PAR-Q (Canadian Society for Exercise Physiology, 2002) and the AHA/ACSM Health/Fitness Facility Preparticipation Screening Questionnaire (American College of Sports Medicine, 2006). Those with increased health risks, identified by one of the self-administered surveys, need to have a medical evaluation prior to starting the activity. As discussed later in this chapter, obtaining an "exercise prescription" from a health care provider can even be a positive motivator for many older adults. The following text contains other safety issues that should be considered before starting a physical activity intervention with this population.

Safety Considerations for Older Adult Physical Activity Interventions

Please note that this is *not* intended to be an all-encompassing list. Practitioners should adapt it to fit the needs of their specific programs and locations.

I. Physical Activity Environment

- Where will the activity take place?
- Is the location accessible to those who may have physical limitations?
- Is the equipment safe and stable?
- Is the activity area free of hazards (e.g., loose carpets, obstructions)?
- What are the emergency procedures? Where is the first aid kit?
- Do all supervisors have appropriate credentials and safety training?

II. Preactivity Screening

- What health screening tool will be used?
- Will medical evaluations be required of high-health-risk participants?
- What procedures will be used?

III. Participant Education

Have the participants been educated about the following?

- Appropriate clothing for the activity including supportive nonskid shoes
- Correct posture for the activity
- Correct breathing techniques
- Listening to the body to identify normal reactions to activity (increased heart rate, breathing rate, and sweating) versus unhealthy reactions (severe shortness of breath, chest pain, joint inflammation, sharp pain)
- Stopping if they encounter pain
- Working within their own limits
- Activity progressions and modifications
- The importance of hydration and how to maintain it

Because the majority of older adults clearly can engage in physical activity safely, a growing body of research has been conducted to identify effective programs for increasing physical activity in this population (Brawley, Rejeski, & King, 2003; Taylor et al., 2004; U.S. Department of Health and Human Services, 1996). However, increasing older adult physical activity participation presents unique challenges. Although some programs have been effective in the short term, the effectiveness of long-term physical activity programs has been limited (Brawley, Rejeski, & King, 2003; Taylor et al., 2004). In an effort to analyze effective methods for increasing physical activity in the older adult population, this chapter will concentrate on the following:

- Identifying factors related to successful older adult physical activity interventions
- Summarizing barriers to physical activity and strategies for overcoming those barriers
- Identifying interventions that have been successful

Factors Related to Successful Physical Activity Interventions

To develop effective older adult physical activity interventions, it is important to understand factors that predict participation and adherence. Numerous research studies have investigated correlates of older adult physical activity participation (Benjamin, Edwards, & Baharti, 2005; Brassington, Atienza, Perczek, DiLorenzo, & King 2002; Hays & Clark, 1999; Lee & Lafferty, 2006; Stuart, Marret, Kelly, & Nelson, 2002). Although many factors influence the participation rates of older adults, we will examine the following, which demonstrate the greatest potential for increasing physical activity:

- Psychological factors of self-efficacy, self-regulation, positive attitudes toward physical activity, and social support
- Health care provider referral
- Physical activity intensity
- Group- and home-based interventions
- Disease management

Psychological Factors

As with other populations, self-efficacy, or the confidence a person has to perform an activity, is one of the strongest determinants of physical activity for older adults (Brassington et al., 2002; Resnick, Orwig, Magaziner, & Wynne, 2002; Schutzer & Graves, 2004). Interventions should help older adults build their confidence through mastery of the physical activity. This can be achieved by beginning the intervention at a low intensity and gradually increasing the intensity over time. This gradual increase is especially important for frail older adults. Improvements in fitness and or health that result from physical activity will also enhance self-efficacy.

To promote long-term adherence to physical activity, interventions need to be designed so older adults move from a supervised, or center-based, setting to the home, where they can use self-regulation skills to make physical activity part of their lifestyle (Rejeski & Brawley, 2006). Behavioral counseling is one method that can be used to help older adults transition from center-based to home-based activity. Through counseling, older adults can develop a plan of action for making physical activity a part of their daily routine.

Having a positive attitude toward physical activity is another factor influencing older adult participation (Stuart et al., 2002). If the activity is positive and enjoyable, older adults will be more likely to continue to exercise. Past participation is also a predictor of future participation (Benjamin et al., 2005). For those who have had a negative attitude toward physical activity, strategies such as providing positive images depicting the activity with role models who may have similar limitations can be used to entice older adults to participate.

Receiving positive reinforcement or social support from friends and family is also one of the predictors of physical activity involvement in the older adult population (Booth, Owen, Bauman, Clavisi, & Leslie 2002; McAuley, Jerome, Elavvsky, Marquez, & Ramsey, 2003; Resnick et al., 2002). Litt, Kepplinger, and Judge (2002) found that social support is a strong determinant of physical activity particularly for older women. In addition, positive comments help strengthen people's self-efficacy and can enhance exercise adherence. Programs need to be carefully designed to create a positive environment. In residential care facilities, older adults may have limited contact with family members; thus, support from friends may be more important.

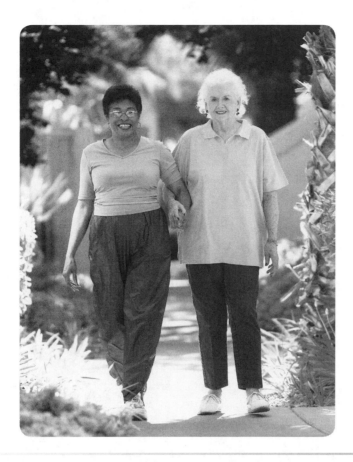

Social support for older adults is a strong determinant of older adults' participation in physical activity programs.

Health Care Provider Referrals

Receiving a recommendation from a physician to exercise is another important positive predictor of physical activity in the older adult population (Benjamin et al., 2005; Navarro, Sanz, del Castillo, Izquierdo, & Rodriguez, 2007; Stuart et al., 2002). Having a health care provider "prescribe" exercise helps older adults overcome their fear of being injured during the physical activity. This type of prescription may be especially important for physically frail older adults (Benjamin et al., 2005). More research needs to be conducted in this area to determine the most effective type of physician advice and the amount of contact needed with the older adult to improve physical activity levels.

Physical Activity Intensity

Older adults are more likely to participate in low- to moderate-intensity physical activity (Brawley et al., 2003; Taylor et al., 2004) such as light housework, chair exercises, and walking. Lower-intensity activity is less likely to

AVRIL ROBARTS LRC

cause injuries and is often perceived as less threatening, especially to older adults who have functional disabilities or limitations. Although interventions should to be tailored to the ability level of the participant, planners must also recognize that low-intensity exercises conducted in a chair may have few functional benefits for the older adult. Specificity of the exercise is the issue. If the goal is to improve mobility and balance, exercises should be conducted while participants are standing and walking. Physical activity interventions that begin at lower intensities should progress over time to moderate intensities.

Group- and Home-Based Interventions

Physical activity interventions can be designed to be group based, home based, or a combination of both. Group-based interventions require participants to go to a facility or center where the activity program is usually supervised. For typical home-based interventions, the physical activity occurs at the older adult's home, and contact with the practitioner is minimal. Combination designs usually begin with a few weeks of group-based instruction followed by a period of home-based activity. Table 6.1 lists some of the positive and negative aspects of group- and home-based interventions.

Research has demonstrated that both home-based and group-based physical activity interventions can be successful with the older adult population (Campbell, Robertson, Gardner, Norton, & Buchner, 1999; King, Haskell, Taylor, Kraemer, & Debusk, 1991; King, Haskell, Young, Oka, & Stefanic, 1995; McMurdo & Rennie, 1993; van der Bij, Laurant, & Wensing, 2002). One study found similar participation rates in both home- and group-based environments for short-term programs; however, adherence rates tended to decrease as the length of the study increased (King et al., 1995; van der Bij et al., 2002). The use of behavioral strategies including phone calls and various incentives may help improve long-term participation rates. More research should be conducted

TABLE 6.1 **Attributes of Group- and Home-Based Physical Activity Interventions**

Type of intervention	Positives	Negatives
Group based	• Activity instruction • Social support • Safety can be monitored	• Classes typically end or take breaks • Participants may not become self-regulating • Transportation issues
Home based	• Easy scheduling • Inexpensive • No pressure to keep pace with others	• Exercises may be done incorrectly • Motivation to be active may be limited • Safety concerns

using a combination of group- and home-based environments to determine which programs work best for which population.

Disease Management

Disease management, in the context of this chapter, is using physical activity as a strategy to prevent disease and maintain favorable health status. Studies have found that mobile older adults who have few or no limitations view physical activity as a way to maintain their health (Cohen-Mansfield, Marx, & Guralnick, 2003; Rasinaho, Herninalo, Leinonen, Linutenen, & Rantinen, 2006). Older adults with higher self-efficacy and a motivation to improve their health are more likely to be physically active than those with lower self-efficacy and little motivation to improve their health (Lee & Lafferty, 2006). Increased self-efficacy may help older adults overcome barriers that prevent them from engaging in physical activity. Physical activity can help all adults, both the young and the old, avoid chronic diseases.

When planning physical activity interventions for older adults, planners should consider factors that will improve participation and adherence. This section highlighted just a few of the factors that typically result in success. Intervention specialists are encouraged to use these strategies to overcome barriers to physical activity in older adults.

Barriers to Physical Activity and Strategies for Overcoming Them

To create successful interventions for older adults, program designers should identify barriers that prevent them from participating in regular physical activity. Figure 6.1 is a checklist that could be used to identify physical activity barriers that older adults may have.

Once intervention specialists understand barriers, they are in a position to develop strategies to address them. Barriers to physical activity, as described in previous chapters, are divided into three categories: personal, environmental, and social. In the older adult population, common personal barriers to physical activity include fear of injury or falling, inertia, and negative past experiences (Rasinaho et al., 2006). Environmental barriers for the older adult include lack of accessibility to facilities or recreational areas and unsafe neighborhoods. Lack of support is viewed as a common social barrier to physical activity.

A strategy for overcoming pain during physical activity (a personal barrier) would be to extend the warm-up period, gently stretch, improve the range of motion in the affected area, and begin the physical activity at a low intensity. If poor access (an environmental barrier) is the issue, one strategy would be to establish the physical activity program in local churches or community centers. Another strategy would be to pair older adults who do drive with those who are unable to drive. Such pairings can also build social support. Table 6.2

Potential Barriers

Please place a check mark next to the barriers that interfere with your ability to take part in regular physical activity.

Personal Barriers

____ Poor health

____ Fear of injury

____ Fear of falling

____ Pain

____ Arthritis pain

____ Lack of knowledge about the benefits of physical activity

____ Being uncomfortable exercising around others

____ Fear of failure

____ Negative exercise experience

____ Other:_____

____ Other:_____

Environmental Barriers

____ Limited funds

____ Difficult access to exercise location

____ No transportation

____ Unsafe neighborhood

____ Bad weather conditions

____ Other:_____

____ Other:_____

Social Barriers

____ Family demands

____ Lack of support from family or friends

____ Other:_____

____ Other:_____

Top Three Barriers

Please identify the top three barriers that might prevent you from being active.

1. _____

2. _____

3. _____

(continued) ▶

FIGURE 6.1 **Questionnaire for identifying older adults' barriers to physical activity and brainstorming solutions to overcome them.**

From L. Ransdell, M. Dinger, J. Huberty, and K. Miller, 2009, *Developing Effective Physical Activity Programs* (Champaign, IL: Human Kinetics).

Solutions for Overcoming the Top Three Barriers

Brainstorm strategies that you would be willing to try to overcome your barriers.

1. _____

   _____

   _____

2. _____

   _____

   _____

3. _____

   _____

   _____

FIGURE 6.1   *(continued)*

TABLE 6.2   **Barriers to Physical Activity in Older Adults and Strategies for Overcoming Them**

Barrier	Strategies for overcoming barrier
Personal	
Poor health	• Begin with low-intensity PA and increase gradually • Take frequent breaks • Find positive role models • Learn about the importance of PA for improving or maintaining health
Fear of injury or falling	• Check with your health care provider (e.g., physician) for a "prescription" to exercise • Use support (e.g., back of a stable chair) when needed during PA
Pain	• Extend your warm-up period • Use gentle stretching to improve your range of motion • Modify your activity when needed • Take frequent breaks • Build strength slowly
Arthritis pain	• Learn about the importance of PA for reducing pain and stiffness (if pain lasts more than 1 hour after exercise, you did too much) • During flare-ups, exercise your noninvolved joints
Lack of knowledge about PA benefits	• Talk to your health care provider about PA • Get a referral from a trusted source (e.g., your health care provider)
Poor self-efficacy	• Set realistic goals • Seek out positive feedback • Record improvements • Find exercise groups that can provide support and encouragement

(continued) ▶

TABLE 6.2 *(continued)*

Barrier	Strategies for overcoming barrier
Personal	
Negative exercise experience	• Find activities that are fun • Begin with a low intensity • Monitor and celebrate improvements
Environmental	
Poor access to or unsuitable exercise environment (unsafe neighborhood)	• Seek out PA programs in your local community centers or churches • Exercise in groups or with friends • Find simple PA programs that could be done at home
Weather conditions	Seek out local PA programs in community centers or churches
Social	
Family demands	Make PA part of your family activity
Lack of support or company	• Join a group-based physical activity program • Find an exercise buddy

Based on Lee and Lafferty, 2006; Lees, Clark, Nigg, & Newman, 2005; Rasinaho, Herninalo, Leinonen, Linutenen & Rantinen, 2006.

lists additional strategies for overcoming barriers. To design successful physical activity interventions, practitioners need to pay special attention to the common barriers and plan strategies to address the issues.

Sample Successful Interventions

Along with addressing motivational strategies and barriers to physical activity for the older adult, it is important to examine successful interventions. The purpose of identifying these physical activity programs is to provide practitioners with ideas that can enhance the delivery of their own older adult programming. Included here are a variety of successful interventions that address important aspects associated with improving physical activity levels in the older adult population.

Fitness and Arthritis in Seniors Trial (FAST)

FAST involved a series of studies that examined the effects of physical activity interventions on functional fitness (i.e., physical activities associated with daily living) and arthritis (Ettinger et al., 1997; Messier et al., 2000). Ettinger and colleagues (1997) examined the effects of aerobic exercise on a group of 439 older adults 60 years of age or older with osteoarthritis. Participants were assigned to health education (e.g., attention control), aerobic exercise, or resistance training groups. The intervention groups were facility based for the first 3 months and home based for the last 15 months. Participants completed exercise log books during the home-based portion, received four home visits, and were contacted regularly by phone. Compared to the control group, the aerobic exercise group improved significantly on the disability questionnaire, knee pain, knee flexion strength, timed walk, stair climb and descent, lifting, and car exit. The resistance training group showed significant improvement over the health education group on physical disability, pain, knee flexion strength, timed walk, lifting, and car exit.

Messier and colleagues (2000) reported on the effects of resistance training, aerobic training, or health education on balance using 113 of the FAST participants. Postural sway (i.e., the ability to lean the body in any direction without having to take a step) was significantly better in the resistance and aerobic training groups when compared to the control group.

Adherence rates for the training groups in these two FAST studies (Ettinger et al., 1997; Messier et al., 2000) decreased significantly, from 85% at 3 months to 50% at 18 months. Even with the declines in adherence, the treatments were effective for improving various aspects of function. Both of these studies demonstrate that exercise can improve function and modify common physical activity barriers for older adults. In addition, they provide effective examples of how exercise programs can move from a supervised setting to a home-based setting where self-regulation skill can be developed.

Home-Based Progressive Strength Training

Osteoarthritis is a common ailment that causes pain, reduces functional abilities, and limits physical activity for many older adults. Baker and colleagues (2001) investigated the effectiveness of home-based strength training for improving symptoms of knee osteoarthritis in a group of 46 adults over the age of 55. Participants were randomized into a nutritional education control group or home-based strength training group. The home-based strength group trained for 4 months. Intervention participants received in-home visits twice a week for 3 weeks, one in the 4th week and every other week thereafter. Compared to the control group, the home-based training group significantly improved in strength, pain reduction, physical function, and quality of life. These important gains highlight the need for home-based programs designed to reduce pain and other osteoarthritis symptoms and improve older adult physical function.

Home-Based Intervention for the Physically Frail Older Adult

Perhaps the most challenging group in need of intervention to improve physical function is that of frail older adults. Gill and colleagues (2002) examined the effectiveness of a 12-month home-based exercise program to reduce functional decline in frail older adults. They assigned 188 frail older adults into a control or home-based intervention group. The home-based intervention group received an average of 16 home visits by a physical therapist for the first 6 months and once monthly thereafter. During the in-home visits, physical therapists removed hazards, taught safe methods to enhance activities, and gave exercise instruction. Participants were also provided an exercise calendar to log their activity. When compared to the control group, the intervention group demonstrated significantly lower disability scores. Those who were moderately frail benefited from the intervention, whereas those with severe frailty did not. This study showed the potential that home-based exercise programs can have for improving the functional abilities of moderately frail older adults.

Fit and Firm and Stretch and Flex

Results from these two yearlong interventions were reported in separate articles. King and colleagues (2000) compared the effects of two physical activity programs (Fit and Firm and Stretch and Flex) on physical function and quality of life outcomes in a group of older adults. Brassington and colleagues (2000) examined cognitive and social factors that facilitate exercise adherence in the elderly. The 103 participants were randomized into one of the two treatments, Fit and Firm, which focused on aerobic activities and strength training, and Stretch and Flex, which involved flexibility exercises. Participants were asked to attend two exercise classes per week and exercise twice a week at home. They also received regular telephone counseling

Brassington and colleagues (2000) found that the Fit and Firm program was effective for improving upper-body strength, heart rate response, and perceptions of strength and endurance. Both groups reported a significant reduction in pain levels. Adherence rates, 79% in Fit and Firm and 80% in Stretch and Flex, were high (King et al. 2000). Self-efficacy and outcome expectations were strongly associated with exercise adherence (Brassington et al., 2000). The results of this study demonstrate that physical function and quality of life can be improved in community-based programs. The high adherence rates also suggest that telephone counseling can increase physical activity in the older adult population.

Shaping Active Living in the Elderly (SALE)

SALE used cognitive-behavioral techniques in a group setting in an effort to increase adherence rates in the older adult population. Brawley, Rejeski, and Lutes (2000) randomized 60 older adults into three groups: wait list control, standard physical activity, or group-mediated counseling. The standard physical activity group (SPA) and the group-mediated cognitive-behavioral (GMCB) subjects participated in a center-based walking program in which classes consisted of a half-hour lecture followed by an hour of exercise. The GMCB participants attended an additional half-hour session in which cognitive-behavioral skills were taught and the social interactions of the group were used to promote adherence and commitment to the program. Self-monitoring, goal setting, behavioral strategies, and exercise plans to increase activity time were also developed to help the GMCB participants adopt a healthy lifestyle.

At the end of the treatment period, both intervention groups had higher health-related quality of life and functional scores than the control group. The GMCB group had a higher physical activity frequency level. These findings suggest that physical activity adherence rates can be improved with the older adult population by using social cognitive strategies and group interactions.

Cardiovascular Health and Activity Maintenance Program (CHAMP)

CHAMP used the concepts from the study by Brawley and colleagues (2000) to address issues of physical activity adherence for people who had completed cardiovascular rehabilitation (Rejeski et al., 2003). Rejeski and colleagues (2003) randomized 147 adults (50-80 years of age) who were at high risk for, or who had, cardiovascular disease (CVD) into a traditional program or a group-mediated cognitive-behavioral program (GMCB). The 12-month walking and upper-body strength training program involved 3 months of center-based training, followed by 6 months of home-based training with minimal contact and 3 months with no contact. Those in the GMCB treatment received additional group counseling on techniques to overcome barriers and develop self-regulation skills.

The findings revealed that the GMCB group significantly improved over the traditional exercise program on peak oxygen uptake, mobility, self-efficacy, and self-reported physical activity. This study also found that men had greater exercise adherence than women and that the older adults in the GMCB program had greater adherence levels. These findings suggest that older adult rehabilitation programs that involve physical activity need to add behavioral and cognitive strategies to help develop self-regulation skills.

Walk; Address Pain, Fear, Fatigue During Exercise; Learn About Exercise; Cue by Self-Modeling (WALC)

WALC was designed to address some of the common barriers older adults have relative to physical activity (Resnick, 2002). Twenty sedentary participants were divided into treatment or control groups. The treatment group followed the four phases of the WALC program. They were asked to walk in groups or individually for 20 minutes three times per week for 6 months. The intervention group received regular visits from a practitioner who addressed unpleasant reactions associated with exercise (i.e., addressed pain, fear, fatigue during exercise). This part of the intervention included pain management techniques, relaxation methods, and scheduling of rest and exercise. Those in the treatment groups were given a book about exercise benefits and barriers and received assistance developing short- and long-term goals, planning exercise sessions, and logging their results (i.e., learned about exercise).

When compared to the controls, the treatment group demonstrated significant improvement in exercise behavior, physical activity levels, and self-efficacy expectations. Although the number of participants used in this study was small, the results indicate that physical activity levels can be increased with the sedentary older adult population by using techniques to improve self-efficacy, which can mediate common exercise barriers.

Community Health Activities Model Program for Seniors (CHAMPS II)

CHAMPS II is based on an earlier study (Stewart et al., 1997) that encouraged older adults living in low-income housing to participate in community physical activity programs. CHAMPS II (Stewart et al., 2001) used motivational and cognitive theory techniques to promote increases in physical activity with older adults. The researchers assigned 173 underactive participants into a yearlong physical activity intervention or a wait list control group. Participants in the intervention group were encouraged to select physical activity programs of their choice. Individual planning sessions, group workshops, educational materials, and activity diaries were provided. The individually tailored programs addressed physical activity barriers, motivational techniques, exercise information and options, and readiness to increase activity levels. Compared to the control group, participants in the intervention group demonstrated significant improvements in physical activity and energy expended per week. This lifestyle intervention program, with an individual approach for improving physical activity, may be a method for improving the health of older adults.

Community Exercise Program (CEP)

Because hip fractures in the older adult population are costly and often associated with high mortality rates (Stevens, Corso, Finkelstein, & Miller, 2006), interventions designed to aid hip fracture rehabilitation are needed. Jones, Jakobi, Taylor, Petrella, and Vandervoort (2006) conducted a pilot study to examine the effectiveness of a community exercise program (CEP) for helping older adults recover from hip fractures. Twenty-seven participants were divided into either an exercise program (CEP) or a control group. The intervention group used standing strength and stepping exercises. Compared to the control group, participants in the CEP group reported significantly greater improvements in self-reported physical ability, mobility, balance, and knee extension strength. Although this was only a pilot study, the findings demonstrate the potential for community-based rehabilitation programs for older adults to aid their recovery from hip fractures or other injuries.

New Zealand's Green Prescription

Elley, Kerse, Aarol, and Robinson (2003) examined the effectiveness of a physician-initiated physical activity program on 878 sedentary 40- to 79-year-old adults. They divided the participants into a wait list control group or an intervention group. Those in the intervention group discussed methods for increasing activity with their primary care providers, who then helped them set activity goals in a prescription form. The participants were contacted three times over the next 3 months by exercise specialists who encouraged them and provided advice on exercise. Newsletters containing physical activity information were sent out quarterly to those in the intervention group. When compared to the controls, those in the intervention group significantly increased their physical activity levels and quality of life. This study demonstrated the potential physician recommendations can have for increasing physical activity in older adults.

❏ Plan for safety (e.g., screening tool, health care provider referral).

❏ Educate participants about the health benefits of physical activity.

❏ Begin with a low-intensity physical activity and gradually increase the intensity over time.

❏ Use strategies to enhance self-efficacy and self-regulation (e.g., goal setting, activity planning, feedback, and charting improvements).

❏ Design a positive activity environment by using positive role models and celebrating successes.

❏ Help identify and develop support networks with family, friends, and groups.

GETTING STARTED

Summary

Improving physical activity levels in the older adult population is an important public health issue that needs to be addressed. This chapter addressed common factors that can enhance programming for the older adult along with common barriers that can prevent older adults from becoming physically active. In addition, the chapter included successful interventions that practitioners can use when designing their own programs. Programs that were most successful fostered mastery and enjoyment of activities (to increase self-efficacy), facilitated movement from center-based to home-based programming, emphasized the social benefits of physical activity, used health care referrals, recommended a progression of activity—from moderate intensity to higher intensities, and promoted activity as a strategy for disease management.

LIVERPOOL JOHN MOORES UNIVERSITY
LEARNING SERVICES

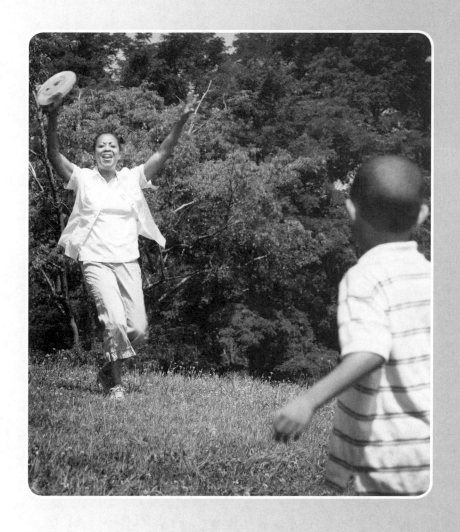

CHAPTER 7

Interventions for Ethnically Diverse Populations

Current statistics suggest that ethnically diverse populations have the highest rates of inactivity in the United States (Centers for Disease Control, 2005). In 1997, the prevalence of sedentary behavior (i.e., no leisure-time physical activity [LTPA]) was as high as 52% in African Americans, 54% in Hispanics, 46% in American Indians/Alaska Natives, and 42% in Asian Americans/Pacific Islanders (Crespo, 2000). One of the goals of *Healthy People 2010* is to decrease the number of U.S. adults who report no LTPA to 20%.

Despite these goals to increase physical activity in minority populations, there are major gaps in the literature that need to be addressed prior to making progress toward this goal (Eyler et al., 1998; Lee, 2005; Marcus et al., 2006). For example, research data related to physical activity participation in African American and Hispanic populations exists; however, little is known about physical activity participation in American Indians/Alaska Natives and Asian Americans/Pacific Islanders (Doshi & Jiles, 2006; Coble & Rhodes, 2006). As with the majority of the population, the potential health benefits of increased physical activity in diverse populations have been documented, and more recently researchers have studied barriers to physical activity in ethnically diverse populations. However, physical activity promotion programs in diverse populations are limited, and few studies have assessed the effectiveness of physical activity interventions that include substantial numbers of racial or ethnic minorities (Lee, 2005; Marcus et al., 2006). These gaps in the literature can make it more difficult to design effective physical activity interventions for minority populations. We reviewed the limited research regarding physical activity in ethnically diverse populations for this chapter with the aim of providing strategies to ensure the successful implementation of physical activity programs with these groups.

Factors Related to Successful Physical Activity Interventions

To create successful interventions, program planners should understand and consider cultural relevancy, some of the social characteristics that define a group's culture, benefits and barriers to physical activity, and how all of these play a role in improving cultural relevancy in the two ethnic groups most prevalent in the United States: Hispanics and African Americans. Specific strategies for cultural relevancy include the following:

■ Recruitment and retention of participants

■ Location of the intervention

■ Delivery of the intervention

The limited literature regarding physical activity interventions and cultural relevancy in American Indian/Alaska Native and Asian American/Pacific Islander populations will also be addressed. Additionally, the few successful studies that have assessed the effectiveness of physical activity promotion in diverse populations will be explored. We recognize that not all people in a particular group are the same; thus, this information is not meant to stereotype. Information provided in this chapter represents a summary of the research literature that is important for health promotion professionals and practitioners to acknowledge and embrace.

Cultural Relevancy and Physical Activity Interventions

Based on the literature, the most important factor in designing and promoting successful physical activity programs for ethnically diverse populations is cultural relevancy (Banks-Wallace & Conn, 2002; Krueter, Lukwago, Bucholtz, Clark, & Sanders-Thompson, 2002; Lee, 2005; Marcus et al., 2006). According to social scientists, culture is learned, shared, and transmitted from generation to generation. To be most effective, physical activity promotion professionals must consider the shared beliefs, norms, values, and practices of the universe of the population (Banks-Wallace & Conn, 2002).

Physical activity promotion professionals must not only consider that certain cultural characteristics may cluster within a given ethnic group, but that substantial differences may exist between individuals and subgroups within populations. For example, familial roles, communication patterns, and spirituality may have commonalities and at the same time be very different. Individual, behavioral, and social characteristics may have special meaning and define a group's culture; ultimately, these cultural factors contribute to the adoption of health behaviors such as physical activity (Krueter et al., 2002).

Social Characteristics and Physical Activity Interventions

Compared to their Caucasian counterparts, minority groups suffer from a disproportionate prevalence of obesity, diabetes, cardiovascular disease, and other chronic diseases that are related to inactivity (Kurian & Cardarelli, 2007; Yancey et al., 2004), thus making the social characteristics of a specific minority group an important factor to consider when trying to implement a successful physical activity program. Specifically, compared to Caucasians, Hispanics have higher rates of diabetes, and African Americans have higher rates of heart disease, stroke, and certain cancers. In fact, 48% of all deaths of African Americans are due to heart disease and cancer (U.S. Department of Health and Human Services [USDHHS], 2003).

In addition to being at a greater risk of chronic diseases related to inactivity, minorities are also more likely to be of low socioeconomic status (SES) and underinsured or uninsured, and more likely to be without activity-promoting resources such as gym memberships, access to safe walking, and personal assistance from health professionals (Albright et al., 2005; Crespo, 2000; Lee, 2005; Whitehorse, Manzano, Baezconde-Garbanati, & Hahn, 1999). Adults with income below the poverty level are three times as likely to be physically inactive as adults in the highest income group (USDHHS, 2003). When physical activity recommendations are met in low-income groups, often their activities are occupational or home-based rather than leisure-related (Ainsworth, Irwin, Addy, Whitt, & Stolarczyk, 1999; Masse et al., 1998). Lower SES is associated with lower physical activity levels (Yancey et al., 2003). The rates of physical inactivity in those without a high school education and an annual family income of less than $10,000 continues to rise compared to the rest of the population (Collins, Lee, Albright, & King, 2004). Underinsured Hispanic women have worse cardiovascular disease (CVD) risk factor profiles than those who are insured (Staten et al., 2004), and African American women of lower SES tend to be more obese than those of higher SES.

The social characteristics of ethnic populations should be a major consideration when designing physical activity programs. It is important to note the problems that exist and how these may affect participation or lack of participation in physical activity when designing intervention programs.

Strategies for Enhancing Cultural Relevancy

Cultural relevancy has to be considered in all physical activity interventions. The shared values, beliefs, and norms of populations affect health behaviors and the likelihood of participating in physical activity interventions. When recruiting and retaining participants, determining the location of the intervention, and delivering the intervention, practitioners should consider cultural relevancy to ensure the success of the physical activity intervention.

Recruitment and Retention

When recruiting diverse populations for physical activity programs, physical activity promotion professionals must first earn credibility in the community. Credibility can be established by developing relationships with community and religious leaders, who can then provide support for a program. For example, church leaders and health care providers trusted in the community can help with increasing recruitment and participation in physical activity interventions. Researchers have suggested that when participants have respect for an individual, they are more likely to participate in the program (Banks-Wallace & Conn, 2002). Community and religious leaders can help PA promotion professionals tap into already existing groups; then, physical activity programs can be implemented and leaders can assist with referring community members to those programs (Yancey, Miles, & Jordan, 1999).

Matching recruitment and retention strategies with the ethnicity of the audience is important. For example, some authors suggest recruiting people from the ethnic group of interest to tell success stories to enhance recruitment and retention (Kreuter et al., 2002; Yancey, McCarthy, & Leslie, 1998). In contrast, some studies don't report ethnicity as a limiting factor for participation, suggesting that it may be more important to have the support of community leaders than a match in ethnicity (Banks-Wallace & Conn, 2002; Yancey et al., 1998).

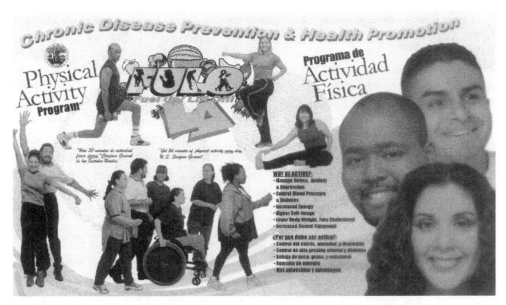

a

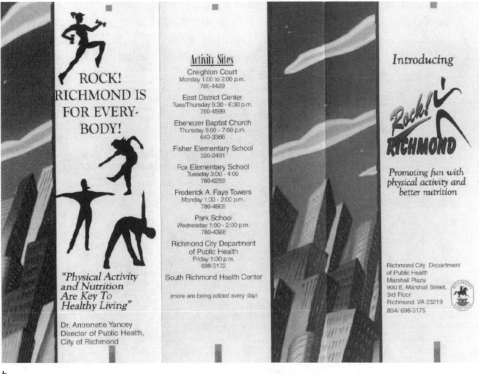

b

Considering the characteristics of the desired audience when designing recruitment materials is vital to a program; it increases potential for subject comfort, trust, and cultural relevance.

Compliments of Dr. Antronette (Toni) Yancy, UCLA and LA County Dept. of Public Health, and Reprinted, by permission, from Richmond Fitness.

Recruitment and retention materials should be distributed specifically for the community. For example, flyers could be mailed to those who subscribe to specific ethnic publications (Chen et al., 1998).

Because language can be a barrier in Hispanic populations, special efforts should be made to advertise in both English and Spanish. Some examples include generating TV spots in Spanish and on Spanish channels, writing newspaper articles that are published in both Hispanic and non-Hispanic papers, and recruiting Spanish speakers to help enroll participants or answer questions (Whitehorse et al., 1999). The colors, images, and fonts of pictures and wording should be relevant to the group of interest (Kreuter et al., 2002). Physical activity programs designed for Hispanics have been successful by using terms such as *Latin dancing* and *Salsa* rather than *aerobics* (Whitehorse et al., 1999). Music should also be tailored to the preferences and interests of the population. Coleman and Gonzalez (2001) were successful in increasing stair use in Hispanics by using culturally relevant signage that was specific to the Hispanic community. Signs were translated and posted in both English and Spanish and had promotional messages for both the individual and the family. Additional recruiting may also be enhanced through presentations at community health fairs, churches, and clinics (Escobar-Chaves, Tortolero, Masse, Watson, & Fulton, 2002).

Research studies have shown that incentives also help recruit and retain people of diverse populations in PA interventions (Banks-Wallace & Conn, 2002; Whitehorse et al., 1999). The incentives, however, should be culturally

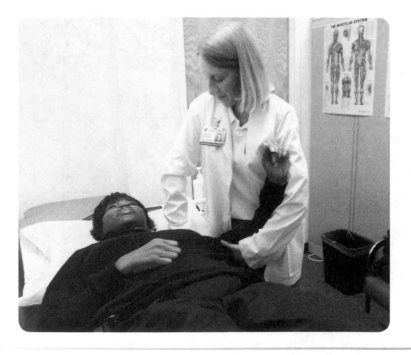

Using incentives, such as a free health screening, can be a crucial part of boosting recruitment in physical activity programs.

appropriate. Community leaders can help PA promotion specialists gather information about the kinds of incentives that would be desirable. Moreover, focus groups with community leaders and members may generate additional incentive ideas. Incentives such as free health screenings, staged monetary payments, certificates of accomplishment, pleasurable experiences such as massages, and T-shirts with the name of the program may help establish an identity among the group and may increase recruitment (Banks-Wallace & Conn, 2002; Escobar-Chaves et al., 2002; Wilbur et al., 2002).

Location of the Intervention

A second component of cultural relevancy is the location or the setting of a physical activity program. A significant part of the lives of both Hispanics and African Americans is the church. Churches have been used to implement a number of physical activity programs in minority communities (Anderson, Wojcik, Winett, & Williams, 2006; Bopp et al., 2006; Lee, 2005; Ransdell & Rehling, 1996; Wilbur, Miller, Chandler, & McDevitt, 2003). Church-sponsored activities such as walking, aerobics, and sports can help to incorporate spirituality, culturally specific activities, and social support within the church and the community, thus increasing physical activity in ethnically diverse populations (Bopp et al., 2006; Yancey et al., 1999).

Delivery of the Intervention

A final component of cultural relevancy is the mode (or method) of delivery. Lee (2005) suggested that physical activity programs should include community collaboration to ensure that they are effective in culturally diverse populations. Physical activity programs should include collaborations among county health departments, local universities, hospitals, and community centers (recreation centers, churches) to strengthen delivery and impact. Partnerships can encourage the pooling of resources to bring down prices for things such as transportation and facilities, which can be major barriers to implementing physical activity programs in diverse populations. Each partner in a collaboration can provide resources according to its strengths; with enough collaborators at the table, barriers to PA can be overcome. The ultimate goal of a community collaboration is to maximize resources.

Personnel for physical activity programs play a large role in the effectiveness of delivering an intervention to ethnically diverse populations. Not only should personnel be professionally trained about how to teach the material and educate the participants, but also, as mentioned in the discussion of recruitment strategies, they should be selected from the community because they are trusted and important members of the community (Banks-Wallace & Conn, 2002; Kreuter et al., 2002). An abundance of literature supports the notion that community personnel should be involved in all aspects of the program from start to finish (design, implementation, evaluation, and interpretation of the findings) (Whitehorse et al., 1999). Additionally, staff should be trained about roles and responsibilities, focus group facilitation and participation, and outreach efforts (Whitehorse et al., 1999; Yancey et al., 1999). A key aspect of WISEWOMAN (Stoddard, Palombo, Troped, Sorensen, & Will, 2004), a cardiovascular disease risk reduction intervention for minority women, was the use of client input for the design and implementation of the program and for the training of all staff in a workshop that focused on innovative outreach and education strategies using cultural competency. With input from the community in the planning stages to ensure the cultural appropriateness of the intervention and greater overall community involvement, it is more likely that the population will feel empowered, excited, and committed to the program (Lee, 2005).

Materials used to deliver the program should also be culturally relevant and packaged to attract a specific group (Kreuter et al., 2002). Visual style can play an important role in helping participants become comfortable and familiar with the material. Moreover, culturally appropriate materials help establish credibility for the program (Kreuter et al., 2002). Health promotion professionals must remember that material must be written in the native language of the population; back translation (i.e., translation from one language to another and then back to the original language, helping to verify the first translation) may be necessary so that the material does not lose its meaning (Coleman & Gonzalez, 2001; Kreuter et al., 2002). As mentioned earlier, the colors, images, and fonts of printed material should appeal to the ethnic population with whom professionals are working.

Finally, because family is highly valued in both African American and Hispanic cultures, physical activity interventions should be designed to nurture family relationships (Banks-Wallace & Conn, 2002). For example, one of the major barriers to physical activity in Hispanic women is gender role constraints. Hispanic women perceive that their time should be spent taking care of the household, working, and being mothers and wives (Heesch & Masse, 2004). Having child care available for little or no charge, or a place where children can play safely while parents are participating in physical activity, may be effective in recruiting and retaining minorities in physical activity interventions (Whitehorse et al., 1999).

Barriers to Physical Activity

Evidence suggests that the major barriers to physical activity in both Hispanics and African Americans are consistent with those of Caucasians. Barriers to physical activity include, but are not limited, to lack of time, motivation, social support, knowledge, health information, transportation, money, and safety (Eyler et al., 1998; Juarbe, Turok, & Perez-Stable, 2002). Although there are similarities among the groups, some barriers are more frequently reported by Hispanics, and others are more frequently reported by African Americans. Table 7.1 lists barriers to physical activity and strategies that can be used to overcome them.

TABLE 7.1   Barriers to Physical Activity in Ethnically Diverse Populations and Strategies for Overcoming Them

Barrier	Strategies for overcoming barrier
Personal	
Lack of knowledge and health information	Seek information about the importance of physical activity, look for programs with tailored or targeted information about physical activity, and competent and educated instructors
Language barriers	Use bilingual education and instructors and translated materials
Environmental	
Transportation	Find programs that are accessible via shuttle service to and from facilities
Money	Look for programs at low- or no-cost facilities (e.g., mall walking groups, physical activity at neighborhood tracks or parks)
Safety	Seek programs that exercise as a group in public areas (e.g., high school tracks, malls, churches)
Social	
Lack of social support from friends, spouse, significant other, family	Find activities for the entire family to participate in together (e.g., church functions), find or develop social networks for women to be active together, learn how to access social support
Lack of role models	Identify active community role models
Gender roles	Seek programs with child care for mothers and gender-specific programs, engage spouse for support

Based on A.A. Eyler, 2002, *Environmental, policy, and cultural factors related to physical activity in a diverse sample of women: The women's cardiovascular health network project* (London, Informa HealthCare).

For example, compared to African Americans, Hispanics more often report lack of time as a contributing factor to inactivity. Additionally, language barriers and gender roles play a part in lack of physical activity participation in Hispanics (Evenson, Sarmiento, Macon, Twaney, & Ammerman, 2002). For example, Hispanic women see child care and family responsibilities as a higher priority than taking care of themselves; this contributes to their perception that there is no time for physical activity. Hispanic women specifically have difficulty enrolling in exercise groups or classes if they don't speak English. Finally, Hispanic women often believe sports are for men, and they don't perceive themselves as able to participate in "sport" activities (Evenson et al., 2002).

Compared to other ethnic minorities and Caucasians, African Americans are more likely to list "lack of safe places to be active" as a major barrier to physical activity (Heesch, Brown, & Blanton, 2000; Juarbe et al., 2002). Specifically, African Americans, particularly those from low SES communities, may fear for their personal safety while being active because of gang member activity or the presence of drug dealers in their neighborhoods (Wilbur et al., 2002). African Americans also frequently report the need for role models who participate in physical activity. African American women have reported that they would look "different" being active in their neighborhood. However, role models may help to increase their self-esteem and make it acceptable to be physically active in their neighborhoods (Wilbur et al., 2002; Young, He, Harris, & Mabry, 2002) Finally, hair maintenance may be a barrier to participation in more vigorous physical activity and longer bouts of physical activity in African American women (Marcus et al., 2006).

Barriers to physical activity within various ethnic populations must be carefully considered when establishing the specific strategies for cultural relevancy and increasing physical activity. Barriers are a major inhibitor to physical activity participation. However, by using designs and strategies that are culturally relevant, barriers can be overcome and physical activity levels can be increased in ethnic populations.

Considerations for Working With Other Diverse Populations

To ensure that physical activity programs are culturally appropriate, promotion professionals must be aware of a group's practices and ways of life. The way in which a group of people live their lives can't be based on identifiable variables such as race (Kreuter, 2001). Differences may exist between groups within populations that may be directly or indirectly related to physical activity behavior. Health promotion professionals must carefully consider this to ensure the success of their physical activity programs.

American Indian/Alaska Native

Little is known about the effectiveness of physical activity interventions in American Indian/Alaska Native (AI/AN) populations. AI/AN have a disproportionate number of health problems compared to Caucasians. According to the Behavioral Risk Factor Surveillance Survey data (Doshi & Giles, 2006), 26.8% of AI/AN women are obese (2001). Additionally, in this population, none of the goals for *Health People 2010* were met relative to smoking, obesity, leisure-time physical activity, or binge drinking (Doshi & Jiles, 2006). AI/AN have a lower life expectancy and higher age-adjusted mortality rate than any other Americans. AI/AN typically have limited access to health care, and many are poverty stricken. The rates of diabetes are much higher in American Indians than in the general U.S. population. For example, in 2002, the prevalence of diabetes in North Carolina was 6.4% in men and 7.9% in women. In comparison, the prevalence of diabetes was 26.9% in AI men and 21% in AI women (Bachar et al., 2006).

Unfortunately, the prevalence of risk factors for health problems in AI/AN populations has received little attention in the health literature (Coble & Rhodes, 2006). In a review of the literature, Coble and Rhodes (2006) discovered that correlates to physical activity were inconsistent and could not be determined because of the lack of literature in the area. Furthermore, there was a gap in information about the models and culturally appropriate methods that could be used to facilitate increased physical activity in American Indians. Younger age, male gender, and high levels of social support were the only factors that were associated with increased physical activity in this ethnic group (Coble & Rhodes, 2006).

Although the effectiveness of culturally relevant physical activity programs in AI/AN populations has not been studied, basic assumptions can be made to begin to design effective interventions for this group. AI/AN have some values that are consistent with other aspects of their culture (Bachar et al., 2006). For example, AI/AN believe in the family unit and the importance of support from all generations. In addition, spirituality for balance is a significant part of an AI/AN lifestyle (Bachar et al., 2006). Therefore, based on studies with African Americans and Hispanics, programs designed for AI/AN should include recruitment, retention, and delivery methods focused on the family. Additionally, physical activity programs for AI/AN may be most effective in recreational or community settings where the whole family can be active with little cost. Finally, considering the strong spirituality practiced amongst most AI/AN, bringing the community together to participate in physical activity may be an important strategy. Belza and colleagues (2006) recommended fostering relationships to positively influence physical activity for all older adult ethnic minority populations, including AI/AN (Belza et al., 2004).

Asian Americans/Pacific Islanders

Asian Americans/Pacific Islanders are another minority population that has been neglected in the health literature. Studies of Asian Americans/Pacific Islanders that address physical activity are sparse (Centers for Disease Control, 2004; Mampilly et al., 2005). Those that have been published often use small sample sizes and combine all Asian American groups, ignoring possible intra-racial differences (Maxwell, Bastani, Vida, & Warda, 2002). Currently there is limited research examining barriers to physical activity participation in this population, and no research assessing what is effective in increasing physical activity. This is very sad considering that the rates of obesity among Pacific Islanders are among the highest in the world (Wang, Abbott, Goodbody, Hui, & Rausch, 1999). Pacific Islanders warrant a very high priority focus as part of public health efforts to address obesity and the relationship between hypokinetic disease and various cardiovascular disease risk factors.

In a qualitative study, Sriskantharajah and Kai (2007) explored the influences on and attitudes toward physical activity in women from South Asia. South Asians have higher rates of death from heart disease and diabetes and are less active than those of European origin. The women from this study were uncertain about the type and level of physical activity in which they should participate. Guidance from their health professionals was lacking, but their motivations and attitudes toward physical activity were similar to those of the general population (e.g., wanting to lose weight, socialize, and maintain independence).

Despite the lack of research with Asian Americans/Pacific Islanders, the necessity for cultural relevancy when designing effective physical activity programs still exists. Program designers can begin to design programs based on a knowledge of other ethnic populations, keeping in mind the need to make culturally relevant changes specific to the population.

Sample Successful Interventions

Even though few studies have specifically assessed the effectiveness of physical activity promotion interventions in racial or ethnic minorities, a limited number of studies exists that can be used as model interventions for minority populations. Four of these model programs are described in the following sections.

WISEWOMAN

As mentioned in chapter 4 (see page 44), WISEWOMAN (Well-Integrated Screening and Evaluation for Women Across the Nation) was designed to decrease risk factors for cardiovascular disease in uninsured and underinsured women over 50 years of age (Stoddard et al., 2004). Specifically, in the Arizona WISEWOMAN project, provider counseling, health education, and community health workers were used to target chronic disease risk factors in uninsured and underinsured Hispanic women over age 50 (Staten et al., 2004). Hispanic women were enrolled from clinics where more than 50% of clients were Hispanic women. The community health workers were trained to provide outreach, translation services, and transportation. The importance of the Arizona WISEWOMAN study was that the community health workers were bilingual, Hispanic, and over 50 years of age. Placing importance on the qualifications of the staff as they relate to the specific ethnic population is essential to implementing successful physical activity programs in diverse populations. All participants of the Arizona WISEWOMAN project significantly increased the number of minutes of moderate-to-vigorous physical activity over 1 year.

Project Walk

Project Walk (Chen et al., 1998) was a home-based phone and mail intervention designed to promote walking in sedentary ethnic minority women. Participants were recruited via presentations at Women, Infants, and Children (WIC) meetings, mailings to subscribers of ethnic publications, flyers distributed throughout the city, and advertisements in local newspapers. All participants had to speak and be able to read English at a sixth-grade level to participate. Women were randomly assigned to one of two conditions: behavioral and educational. Phone calls were made to all participants; however, those who were in the educational comparison condition didn't receive any behavioral counseling or extensive discussion over the phone. Instead, they were offered a 5-minute call in which program recommendations for walking were presented. The behavioral condition received six telephone counseling sessions. Both groups had substantial increases in minutes walked (Chen et al., 1998). Project Walk was successful in encouraging both Hispanics and African Americans to engage in physical activity.

impACT

The impACT (Increasing Motivation for Physical ACTivity) project (Albright et al., 2005), also mentioned on pages 44-45, was an intervention designed to determine the difference between personalized behavioral skills counseling and print materials relative to the initiation and maintenance of physical activity in low-income ethnic minority women, some of whom were unemployed. Classes were 1 hour a week for 8 weeks and were designed to motivate women to become physically active through behavior skills such as overcoming barriers, setting goals, and developing a personal physical activity program. The classes were also culturally sensitive for the Latina population. For example, the health educators were ethnically matched and gave the women guidance about how to be active and respect their core values (e.g., go walking during lunch so that it doesn't interrupt evening responsibilities).

After the initial 2 months, women were randomized to a home-based group that either received print materials or received print materials in addition to phone counseling. Women who were in the print materials plus phone counseling group significantly increased their physical activity and maintained their activity over 10 months (Albright et al., 2005). This program provides another good example of using culturally tailored education and behavior skills to increase physical activity in minority populations.

La Vida Caminando

La Vida Caminando (Grassi, Gonzalez, Tello, & He, 1999) was a community physical activity intervention that was designed by and for Latino families residing in rural cities in central California. The purpose of this study was to promote regular, moderate physical activity in accordance with recommendations from the Centers for Disease Control. The objectives of the program were to (a) add at least one new physical activity resource within each of the four communities; (b) involve at least 200 adults in walking clubs to engage them in a minimum of 30 minutes of walking, three times a week, for at least 3 months; and (c) organize other community-based activities and events to increase awareness of the benefits of physical activity involving at least 100 community members. Local advisory committees were formed that identified priorities such as that the physical activity programs be low cost, low impact, and family friendly, and that they include Spanish (both spoken and used in materials) and diabetes and weight management education.

The walking clubs had attendance ranging from 8 to 35 participants, and walks included physical activity training and discussions about healthy nutrition and other ways to reduce the risk of chronic disease. All participants were interviewed when they joined the club, at 6 months, and at 1 year. The interview was a face-to-face self-report or telephone self-report about demographics, activity type and frequency, and barriers.

Physical activity decreased from baseline to 6 months (7.5-12.9 hours per week to 3.0-6.2 hours per week). There were no changes in physical activity from 6 months to 1 year. Despite the decrease in physical activity, there were decreases in barriers reported between 6 months and 1 year. The following barriers decreased during the intervention: *no nearby location for physical activity, unsafe neighborhood, lack of transportation, high cost (unaffordable), not knowing where to go for physical activity,* and *not knowing how to start a physical activity program.* Two barriers to physical activity that increased over the year were *family responsibility* and *work schedule.* Health problems did not change over time, and language was not a barrier (Grassi et al., 1999). Although there were no increases in physical activity over the year, this program is a good example of using the community to decrease barriers to physical activity as well as a great example of designing programs with the community for the community.

GETTING STARTED

❑ Earn credibility with community and religious leaders.

❑ Build collaborations within the community to maximize resources.

❑ Advertise using words, pictures, fonts, and messages that are culturally relevant.

❑ Translate messages without losing the meaning of the message.

❑ Use personnel of matching ethnicity as role models to recruit for and deliver the intervention whenever possible.

❑ Build on or from already existing groups to recruit participants.

❑ Get input from community personnel about all aspects of the program.

❑ Facilitate focus groups with community leaders and community participants.

❑ Offer culturally relevant incentives.

❑ Offer programs in churches or community settings.

❑ Include the family and extended family in program activities.

❑ Provide child care for parents whenever possible.

Summary

The "Getting Started" checklist includes a summary of the most important aspects to consider prior to implementing a program. To design effective physical activity interventions for ethnically diverse populations, program designers must consider the social characteristics, barriers to physical activity, and cultural relevancy of each population. Strategies for recruitment and retention of participants, the location of the intervention, and how the intervention is delivered must be in line with the culture of the population. This will help to ensure the success of a program, which includes increasing physical activity. Considering the lack of research on minority populations and the growing obesity (and hypokinetic disease) epidemic disproportionately affecting minorities, there is a dire need to continue to design, implement, and evaluate effective physical activity programs for ethnic populations.

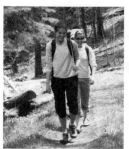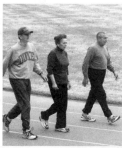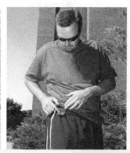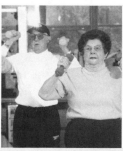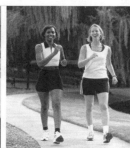

Considering the Variables

This book has covered a lot of territory related to developing effective physical activity interventions. Part I laid the foundation by presenting crucial information to help guide the planning process. Part II identified key considerations related to working with specific populations. This third and final part expands on the groundwork laid in the previous parts and challenges intervention developers to take into account how the environment, the setting, and the use of technology influence intervention planning.

Chapter 8 focuses on the built environment and the many ways neighborhood and community design influence physical activity. Chapter 9 provides insight into the variety of settings in which physical activity interventions take place—the home, the family, the church, the medical community, and the worksite. Chapter 10 addresses the ever-increasing opportunities to take advantage of technology and deliver interventions in ways other than face-to-face. This is known as mediated program

PART

three

delivery, and it uses mass media, print, phone, and Web-based approaches to positively affect physical activity levels.

We hope this book has accomplished its purpose of addressing issues relevant to populations that would most benefit from increasing physical activity. Moreover, it has been our desire to assist intervention developers in their efforts to enhance the quality of life of those they serve.

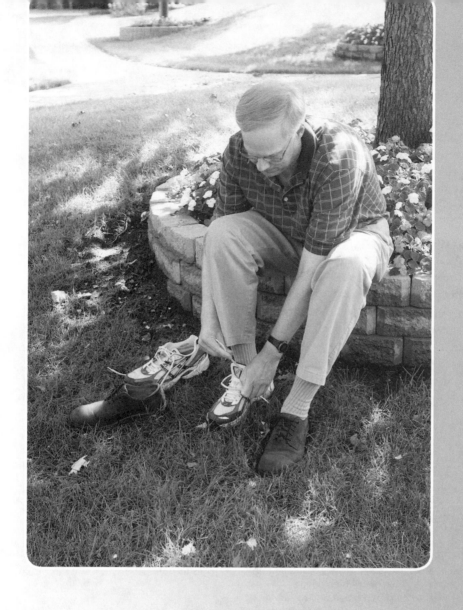

CHAPTER 8

Increasing Physical Activity Through Environmental Approaches

Traditionally, theoretical approaches to changing health behaviors have focused on the individual level, attempting to encourage and empower people to engage in healthier lifestyles. This approach has been effective in some ways, but we know that people in the United States still do not engage in enough physical activity to maintain good health. Some researchers have developed an ecological framework as a means to understanding the multiple influences on health behavior. The ecological framework identifies intrapersonal, interpersonal, environmental, and policy influences on behavior (Sallis & Owen, 1997). This chapter addresses the third construct in the framework: environmental influences, specifically the built environment. The term *built environment* refers to transportation and land development patterns as well as neighborhood design (Cunningham & Michael, 2004). Table 8.1 provides definitions of elements related to the built environment and how they affect physical activity.

One of the *Healthy People 2010* objectives is to increase opportunities for physical activity through "creating and enhancing access to places and facilities where people can be physically active" (U.S. Department of Health and Human Services, 2000). This objective is relevant in today's world because

TABLE 8.1 **Definitions of Terms Related to Components of the Built Environment**

Term	Definition	Why it matters
Street connectivity	The ease of travel between two points. The degree to which streets or areas are interconnected and easily accessible to one another. An example of high connectivity would be a dense grid pattern in a downtown area.	Makes walking and biking easier by providing direct routes to destinations
Safety	The presence or absence of unleashed dogs, perceived threat of physical harm, presence of streetlights.	People must feel safe in order to be comfortable being active outdoors
Open space	A part of the countryside not developed and reserved for recreational or similar purposes.	Provides opportunities for physical activity
Density	The compactness of development. Common measures of density include population per acre or square mile and dwelling units per acre.	People living in more densely populated areas tend to engage in more walking and physical activity
Mixed use	Juxtaposition of land classifications, such as residential, office, commercial, industrial, park, and flood plain within a given area. Land use is controlled by zoning ordinances that reflect political decisions often made at the local level.	Encourages people to walk rather than drive to conduct business
New urbanism	Design trend that mimics the way neighborhoods and communities were built when residences and commerce were organized around a central point rather than spread out.	Encourages people to walk rather than drive to conduct business and promotes a greater sense of community

with increased reliance on technology, people are less physically active in their daily lives. Activity has been engineered out of the lives of most Americans. Unfortunately, many Americans are not motivated to engage in purposeful exercise. For this reason, one approach to increasing activity levels is to create environments that are conducive to incorporating at least moderate physical activity into our lives.

This chapter describes several approaches and issues related to the influence of the environment on physical activity. The following aspects of the built environment that can affect physical activity are addressed:

- Interventions to increase stair use
- Impact of neighborhood design
- Presence of trails and parks
- Ways the environment influences people's physical activity based on socioeconomic and demographic factors
- Environmental assessment tools and other resources for practitioners

Stairwell Interventions

Early recommendations for physical activity proved to be difficult for many people to attain and thus were not effective in increasing physical activity for the average person. Activity recommendations were later revised to support the value of 30 minutes of moderate activity that could be achieved through several bouts throughout the day (American College of Sports Medicine, 1998). With this change in philosophy, it became clear that it was possible to improve health through some activities of everyday life, such as using stairs rather than elevators or escalators. The Centers for Disease Control and Prevention (CDC) developed an intervention designed to encourage people to use the stairs as an alternative to using an elevator or escalator. The StairWELL to Better Health intervention began with a study in 1998 to determine whether improving the appearance and usability of stairwells might increase usage (Centers for Disease Control and Prevention [CDC], 2007). Physical changes such as playing music, displaying motivational signs, and enhancing the overall aesthetics of the stairwell were made, and researchers observed the number of people who used the stairwell. The intervention was successful in encouraging more people to use the stairs than had used them prior to the study. When researchers discovered that improving the appearance of stairs could actually increase the number of people who used them, the CDC then developed guidelines so others might develop similar interventions to increase stair usage in their buildings.

Signs

According to the CDC, using the StairWELL intervention can help people develop a healthy new habit with point-of-decision prompts in the form of motivational signs (CDC, 2007). There are four major things to consider when developing such signs. First, the messages conveyed on the signs should be appropriate for the demographic group that is most likely to read them. For example, if the signs are intended for an older population, it would be valuable to include some reference to the impact of stair climbing on cardiovascular health, whereas for a younger population for whom CVD is often not a pressing issue, an emphasis on weight control might be more effective. Second, some researchers (Webb & Eves, 2007) found that simple messages focused on the specific outcomes to be gained by taking the stairs may be more effective than more general motivational messages. Thus, although "Hey, thought about the stairs?" or "No time to exercise today? Your opportunity is now!" may influence some, messages such as "Stair climbing burns 100 more calories than using the elevator" or "Stair climbing is healthy for your heart" are more likely to be effective because they are more specific. The CDC provides several examples of messages that could be used to facilitate increased stair usage (www.cdc.gov/nccdphp/dnpa/hwi/toolkits/stairwell/motivational_signs.htm#Message%20Ideas). Third, the credibility of the messages is important (Webb & Eves, 2007). Those who read the messages need to be convinced that the information is accurate. To increase the likelihood of message credibility, it would be helpful to have a known physician or celebrity endorse the messages, or to provide a credible source for each message. Finally, if sign usage is being considered as part of an intervention to increase stair usage, it is important to pilot test signs with a group similar to that being targeted in the intervention. Pilot testing can be done with focus groups or simply by asking people informally what they think about the signs. Sample signs are available at the CDC Web site (www.cdc.gov/nccdphp/dnpa/hwi/toolkits/stairwell/motivational_signs.htm#Message%20Ideas).

Stairwell Appearance and Aesthetics

Stairways are often designed strictly for utilitarian purposes with little concern for aesthetics. Improving the appearance of stairwells can positively affect people's willingness to use stairs. In the CDC's intervention, stairs were carpeted and rubber treading was added for safety. Walls were painted a pleasing color, artwork was installed, and music was broadcast. Motivational signs were also included in the stairwells. Results from a study conducted by Boutelle, Jeffery, Murray, and Schmitz (2001) supported the value of improving the aesthetics of stairwells. In their study comparing the effectiveness of motivational signs alone versus signs along with music and artwork, the addition of music and artwork significantly increased stair use. In other words, improving the aesthetic quality of the stairs increased usage.

It may not be possible to incorporate all of these changes in a given building because of codes that may be in place, but it is worthwhile to examine the potential for even minor changes if they promote increased physical activity. As with other aspects of this type of intervention, the CDC Web site provides guidelines for how to begin improving the appearance of a stairwell (www.cdc.gov/nccdphp/dnpa/hwi/toolkits/stairwell/other_ideas.htm).

Tracking and Other Issues

Depending on the objectives of the intervention, it might be valuable to implement some type of tracking system to determine whether the intervention was effective. A very simple way to accomplish this is to have observers count the number of people who use the stairs over a given period of time—prior to and after the intervention. It may also be helpful to conduct this simple evaluation at various times such as immediately before, immediately after, a few months after, and 1 year after the intervention, to know whether the changes were maintained over time. New technologies are being created to more accurately measure foot traffic, but these will probably be more expensive at the onset compared to direct observation.

Neighborhood Design

The relationship between physical activity and neighborhood design has been studied fairly extensively in recent years (Berrigan & Troiano, 2002; Brownson, Baker, Houseman, Brennan, & Bacak, 2001; Craig, Brownson, Cragg, & Dunn, 2002; Ewing, Schmid, Killingsworth, Zlot, & Raudenbush, 2003; Moudon & Drewnowski, 2005; Sharpe, Granner, Hutto, & Ainsworth, 2004). The majority of studies are cross-sectional and draw conclusions based on associations between characteristics of neighborhoods and the physical activity behaviors of its residents. At this point, very few intervention studies have been conducted—mainly due to logistical reasons. Therefore, conclusions from the research discussed in this section are limited as a result of the paucity of research. Nevertheless, some strong associations have been found between certain neighborhood characteristics and physical activity. Specifically, some aspects of neighborhood design that are related to physical activity are neighborhood age and design, proximity to services, aesthetics, and walkability.

Neighborhood Age and Aesthetics

In a unique study, Berrigan and Troiano (2002) analyzed data from the Third National Health and Nutrition Examination Survey (NHANES III) to examine the association between the age of homes in multiple neighborhoods and the walking behaviors of residents of those neighborhoods. The researchers found that those who lived in older homes in older neighborhoods were more likely to walk 1 or more miles (1.6 km or more) at least 20 times per month. An "older home" was defined as having been built before 1973, according to the researchers. Neighborhoods and homes built during this time period are closer together and the streets tend to be laid out in a gridlike pattern (i.e., street connectivity) without cul-de-sacs and with shorter block lengths. In addition, there is often a mix of homes and businesses such as restaurants, grocery stores, and markets that provide a destination for walking trips. This relationship between the age of homes and walking behaviors was found in urban and suburban homes but not in rural homes. The age of the home was not associated with the walking behaviors of rural residents.

The attractiveness of a neighborhood is also associated with overall activity and with recreational walking (Brownson et al., 2001; Craig et al., 2002; Giles-Corti et al., 2005; Handy, Cao, & Mokhtarian, 2006). An attractive neighborhood is one that includes pleasant scenery and has an inviting, safe atmosphere. The perception of what is aesthetic may vary from person to person, and it is unclear specifically what characteristics positively influence walking in a neighborhood. More research is needed to more closely define the neighborhood characteristics most associated with physical activity.

In another interesting study, Ewing and colleagues (2003) found that people living in the most densely populated areas of the United States were less likely to be obese and hypertensive. For example, residents of New York County were less likely to be obese and hypertensive than residents of a much less densely populated suburban county in Ohio in which there is a great deal of sprawl (i.e., homes and businesses are much more spread out and require more car travel compared to more densely populated areas). It is possible that people who live in densely populated places engage in more physical activity as part of daily living because it is simply more convenient to walk or take public transportation than to drive. Having a car and traveling by car in crowded cities is much less convenient and more expensive than walking or using public transportation. Craig and colleagues (2002) studied the interactions among several demographic variables, the environment, and physical activity in several communities in Canada. They found that those in urban areas were more likely to use public transportation or walk or bike to work compared to those in suburban areas.

Walkability

What makes a neighborhood walkable, or supportive of overall physical activity? The presence of sidewalks in good condition, social and community support for walking, streetlights, and access to places and opportunities for physical activity are all positively associated with walking and other forms of physical activity. Several studies have found relationships between sidewalks and various types of physical activity (Sharpe et al., 2004). Seeing others walking and exercising in the neighborhood positively influences residents to engage in physical activity. Streetlights in good working order (Troped, Saunders, Pate, Reininger, & Addy, 2003) are also associated with greater levels of walking and physical activity. This is not surprising given that people need to feel safe before they will engage in outdoor activities.

Another important part of a walkable neighborhood is the presence of services close to where people live. Having grocery stores, restaurants (other than fast food), bars, and taverns, and retail establishments within walking distance increases the likelihood of walking for transportation. This type of land use is more typically found in urban settings than in suburban or rural settings.

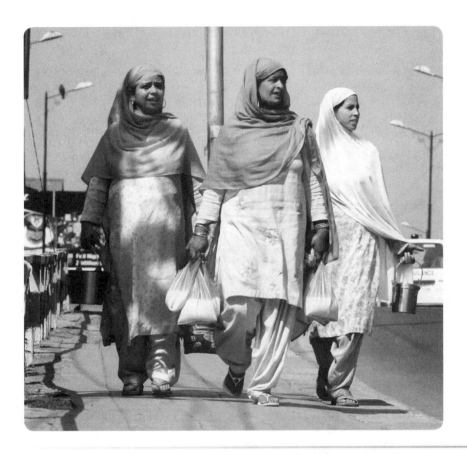

Having grocery stores and other services within waling distance increases the liklihood of walking for transportation.

As the preceding discussion demonstrates, a great deal of evidence suggests that neighborhood design plays an important role in influencing the physical activity behaviors of residents.

Trails and Parks

Findings from research on the impact of trails and parks on physical activity are varied partly because of differences in study design. Many cross-sectional studies show associations between the presence of trails and parks and higher activity levels of those living near them (Addy et al., 2004; Giles-Corti et al., 2005; Gordon-Larsen, Nelson, Page, & Popkin, 2006; Huston, Evenson, Bors, & Gizlice, 2003). However, other studies conducted before and after such outdoor facilities were created have shown different outcomes. Evenson, Herring, and Huston (2005) conducted telephone surveys with residents living close to a trail before and after trail installation. Researchers found no increase in physical activity after the trail installation among adults living near the trail.

In an attempt to increase trail use, Brownson, Baker, and colleagues (2004) conducted interventions in communities that developed walking trails and found that they were able to increase residents' trail use, but the more general impact of trail use on overall physical activity was not changed. In other words, it may be that people who were already physically active used the trails, but they did not become more active as a result of using the trails.

The Robert Wood Johnson Foundation (2007) recently published a synthesis of research conducted on the impact of trails and parks on physical activity. They reported that "Parks and open spaces are associated with walking for transportation but not with recreational walking" (p. 6). This finding is unexpected, but there may be a logical explanation. The availability of trails and parks may not influence those who are already physically active; however, trails and parks may provide opportunities to walk for transportation that were not previously present. If this is the case, then it is still beneficial to provide trails and parks because they bring opportunities for physically active transportation that may not have previously existed. As with other aspects of research related to the impact of the environment on physical activity, it is difficult to come to definitive conclusions because studies are fairly few and study designs tend to be cross-sectional. Therefore, a cause-and-effect relationship is difficult to establish.

Socioeconomic Status and Demographic Considerations

Much of the research on the environmental influences on physical activity has been conducted on middle-class adults. Consequently, little is known about how the environment potentially affects people from economically diverse backgrounds. Similarly, it is unclear whether the environment affects people differently based on gender, age, or race or ethnicity. The research thus far does suggest that differences exist.

An analysis of data from the National Longitudinal Study of Adolescent Health indicated that disparities exist in terms of access to recreational facilities (Gordon-Larsen et al., 2006). Those with lower socioeconomic status (SES) and groups with greater numbers of minorities typically have less access than those with higher SES. At the same time, those in the lower SES group were more likely to be overweight and less likely to engage in physical activity. The higher SES groups tended to have one or more facilities available to them, and this was associated with lower incidence of overweight and higher levels of physical activity (Gordon-Larsen et al., 2006).

Ainsworth, Wilcox, Thompson, Richter, and Henderson (2003) assessed the correlates of physical activity among African American women in South Carolina and found that seeing people exercise in their neighborhood and having sidewalks available were two factors associated with higher levels of physical activity. Light traffic (as opposed to heavier traffic) was shown to be related to physical activity, but this was not a statistically significant relationship. Conversely, Young and Voorhees (2003) studied urban African American women and found no association between physical activity and specific environmental factors.

In general, minorities are more likely to walk for transportation than whites, but they do get less overall activity. The fact that minorities walk more than whites might be due to a lack of cars, but it may also be because many minorities in the United States live in urban environments that are more walkable.

Where people live (e.g., urban, suburban, or rural) may influence the way the environment influences physical activity. Parks, Housemann, and Brownson (2003) reported that, in their cross-sectional study of diverse populations, people in lower SES and living in urban areas were more likely to be physically active if they had access to parks and trails. This pattern was evident among higher SES urban dwellers because access to gyms and exercise equipment increased the likelihood of physical activity; the same was true for lower SES suburban dwellers. Those from lower SES backgrounds living in rural areas were more likely to be physically active if sidewalks were present. Access to gyms was the only environmental factor associated with physical activity among rural residents in higher SES groups.

Very few studies exist on how older populations' physical activity may be affected by their environment. In one study of leisure-time physical activity (LTPA) among rural, middle-aged, and older women, rural women were less likely to be physically active than urban or suburban women. These women were also likely to report that having sidewalks, streetlights, safe places to exercise, access to facilities, and role models (e.g., seeing others who exercise) influenced their activity levels (Wilcox, Castro, King, Housemann, & Brownson, 2000). Cunningham and Michael (2004) reported that perceptions of safety, neighborhood appearance, and living close to services are potentially more important influences on older peoples' activity compared to that of their younger counterparts.

Finally, people may interact uniquely with their environment based on their stage in life. Neighborhood designs that support children's activity (cul-de-sacs with little traffic, more open space) may affect adults in a different way because those characteristics are negatively associated with physical activity among adults. More research needs to be conducted to understand the differences related to life stage.

Instruments to Measure Physical Activity Influences

Researchers examining the relationship between the environment and physical activity have created increasingly sophisticated methods to measure influences and help increase our understanding. Many instruments exist to examine environmental attributes and physical activity. A few are described in the following sections, and others are in development.

Community Audits

Community audits are tools that researchers and practitioners can use to assess the built environment of a community. Brownson, Hoehner, and colleagues (2004) tested the reliability (i.e., whether similar results can be obtained in multiple administrations) of two audit instruments designed to examine walkability and bikability. There were two versions of the audit instruments. One was designed for use during telephone interviews with community residents; it inquired about walking behaviors and perceptions of the environment for walking and physical activity. The phone interview version used a Likert scale with ordinal response choices. A Likert scale asks respondents to indicate the level to which they agree or disagree with given statements, for example, *Strongly Agree, Agree, Neutral, Disagree, Strongly Disagree.* The second audit was a checklist (see figure 8.1) designed to be used by a trained observer to indicate characteristics present in a community. It assessed factors such as the types of buildings (single-family, apartment buildings, mobile homes), land

1. What land uses are present?
   - _____ a. Are residential and nonresidential land uses present?
     - _____ i. All residential
     - _____ ii. Both residential and nonresidential
     - _____ iii. All nonresidential
2. Is public transportation available?
   - _____ a. Are transit stops accessible and visually pleasing?
3. What street characteristics are visible?
   - _____ a. Are there marked lanes?
   - _____ b. Are there medians or pedestrian stands?
   - _____ c. Are there turn lanes?
   - _____ d. Are there crosswalks?
4. What is the quality of the environment?
   - _____ a. Are commercial buildings adjacent to the sidewalks?
   - _____ b. Are there benches, drinking fountains, and other amenities designed for human comfort?
5. Do you have a place to walk or bicycle?
   - _____ a. Are there sidewalks?
     - _____ i. Are they in good condition without breaks or cracks?
   - _____ b. Are there bike lanes?

FIGURE 8.1 **Sample checklist for community audits.**

Adapted from *Journal of Physical Activity and Health,* Vol. 1, R.C. Brownson et al., "Reliability of two instruments for auditing the environment for physical activity," pgs. 191-208, Copyright 2004, with permission from Elsevier.

use, transportation options, and several other characteristics. The researchers found that the instruments were fairly to highly reliable, based on the specific attribute being assessed. In particular, items assessing transportation and land use demonstrated high reliability, and the researchers suggested that those items can be measured with confidence. More specific information and access to both of the versions of the audits can be obtained at www.prc.slu.edu.

Neighborhood Environment Walkability Scale (NEWS)

The NEWS is a written survey developed to provide a comprehensive assessment of a community for walking and other physical activity. Among the neighborhood characteristics included in this assessment are residential density, land use mix, street connectivity, appearance, street design, safety, access to services, and satisfaction with various aspects of a neighborhood (Saelens, Sallis, Black, & Chen, 2003). Subscale scores range from 1 to 4 for most of the subscales, with a few exceptions, and higher scores indicate a more walkable neighborhood. The researchers indicate that the NEWS is reliable and valid. More information about this tool can be found at www.drjamessallis.sdsu.edu/NEWS.pdf.

Geographic Information System (GIS)

Used extensively by geographers, GIS is now being used to study the relationship between physical activity and the environment. GIS creates maps that can integrate data and geographic characteristics (Porter, Kirtland, Neet, Williams, & Ainsworth, 2004). Epidemiologists use GIS as a way to track or identify patterns of disease prevalence in certain areas (e.g., the prevalence of cardiovascular disease in the southeastern United States) or to determine the potential pockets of disease incidence. GIS is an advancement in research on physical activity and the environment because it does not rely on self-report and it can relate physical activity to the actual environment. GIS technology can be costly and requires expertise. Nonetheless, it is very likely that GIS will become a valuable tool in learning more about the relationship between physical activity and the environment.

Other Resources

Many resources exist to assist those interested in improving their community environment for physical activity. The National Center for Biking and Walking Web site (www.bikewalk.org) and Walkable Communities, Inc. (www.walkable.org) are two organizations that provide extensive support for anyone interested in learning more about what makes a community more walkable and bikable. These Web sites are also helpful for those who hope to influence their communities to incorporate designs that support activity.

Another informative source is www.activelivingresources.org, the Web site for the Active Living Resources Center. Its mission is to empower and enable community residents to advocate for making their communities supportive of walking and biking. A final resource is the Smart Growth Network. This is a coalition of nonprofit and government organizations that guide and encourage communities to be mindful of how they plan neighborhoods and how those plans affect the environment and, therefore, the people who live there (www. smartgrowth.org).

GETTING STARTED

❏ Look for ways to incorporate physical activity in activities of daily life such as encouraging using stairs instead of elevators or escalators.

❏ Develop attractive and motivating signs with messages encouraging physical activity.

❏ Identify simple ways to evaluate the effectiveness of environmental interventions on physical activity.

❏ Use a community audit tool to determine whether the environment supports physical activity and is walkable or bikable.

❏ Encourage the use of community trails and parks as venues for physical activity.

❏ Consider issues of diversity when developing interventions to make the environment more supportive of physical activity.

❏ Work to increase awareness among community residents of how the environment influences physical activity.

Summary

This chapter discussed a range of issues related to the relationship of the built environment and physical activity including interventions to increase stair use, the impact of neighborhood design, the presence of trails and parks, socioeconomic and demographic factors, and approaches to measuring the built environment. The body of literature on this topic is growing every day, and a comprehensive review could easily be a book in itself. This is an exciting and challenging time in which our understanding of the influences on physical activity is expanding. The next phase is to learn how to develop interventions to determine the extent to which environments and people interact and how physical activity can be increased on the population level.

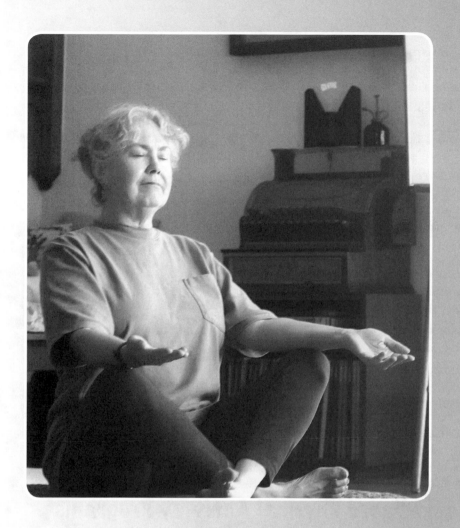

CHAPTER 9

Increasing Physical Activity by Considering the Setting

As compared to the built environment, which is covered in chapter 8, this chapter covers the immediate, existing environment, or setting. The term *setting* refers to the location in which physical activity takes place. For adults, setting may include the home or family, church, medical community, or worksite. Schools are considered a unique setting for physical activity, but because this book targets adult populations, physical activity programming in the school setting is not covered in this chapter. Just as gender, age, and ethnicity may influence participation in physical activity, setting can have a significant impact on whether an individual is physically active. How comfortable a person feels in a specific setting and how convenient that setting is may also affect whether that person engages in activity. Given the importance of setting relative to promoting physical activity, the purpose of this chapter is to do the following:

- Summarize important factors for promoting physical activity in five settings (i.e., home, family, church, medical community, and worksite)
- Discuss setting-specific barriers to activity and some ways to overcome those barriers
- Identify and describe programs that have been successful in the five settings covered in this chapter

The organization of this chapter is somewhat different from that of previous chapters in that all information about one setting will be covered before moving on to the next setting. This will enable physical activity intervention specialists to easily locate information about the setting in which they are working.

Home-Based Physical Activity Programs

Home-based physical activity programs include any programs that can be completed at or near the home. Typically, these programs are simple and include some sort of training session (in person, via the Internet, or via tapes or CDs), and they recommend completing logs of activity and developing specific goals and aims. Ideally, home-based programs should have some sort of leader with whom participants can check in if they experience difficulties. Because of their convenience, these programs are inexpensive and attractive to populations such as women with small children or other caregiving responsibilities, the elderly, low-income people, rural residents, and the diseased or injured (Wilbur, Miller, Chandler, & McDevitt, 2003).

Factors Related to Successful Home-Based Programs

Many home-based physical activity programs were designed by the medical community in an attempt to improve postsurgery recovery (Carmeli, Sheklow, & Coleman, 2006; Keays, Bullock-Saxton, Newcombe, & Bullock, 2006; Pinto, Frierson, Rabin, Trunzo, & Marcus, 2005) or an existing health problem (Mayoux-Benhamou et al., 2005; Petrella & Bartha, 2000; Tuzin et al., 1998; Zion, De Meersman, Diamond, & Bloomfield, 2003). Other programs were designed to prevent hypokinetic disease or improve quality of life in predominately healthy populations (Leaf & Reuben, 1996; Taggart, Taggart, & Siedentop, 1986) or test the cost-benefit ratio of a home-based program in an increasingly expensive medical care system (Robertson, Devlin, Gardner, & Campbell, 2001). Regardless of the purpose of a home-based program, factors related to success in such programs are similar. These factors are summarized in the following list.

▪ *Provide training sessions.* The essentials for successfully completing training should be described in a training session (or sessions) that occurs prior to the home-based activity sessions. Training sessions should be conveniently located for participants, either at their homes or at a centrally located activity site. Providing participants with basic education about what they are supposed to do will increase their confidence and motivation to try a home-based program.

▪ *Provide program details.* Program details (e.g., activity demonstrations, progressions) should be provided via Web link downloads, CDs, videotapes, or DVDs (or all four). Because most people do not like to take time to figure out exercises or activities, they are more likely to follow programs that are simple, easily available, and well explained than those that are complicated, lengthy, or hard to access.

▪ *Ask for a reasonable time commitment.* Physical activity or exercise sessions should be limited to a reasonable period of time. Given that many people participate in home-based activity because of existing time constraints, it is important to design a program that can be completed in 30 to 60 minutes. In all of the home-based programs reviewed for this chapter, none required a time period longer than 60 minutes. Programs that require longer than 60 minutes may have lower levels of compliance than those that require a time period less than 60 minutes.

▪ *Teach participants to negotiate role balance.* When participants are taught how to negotiate role balance (i.e., ways to share household responsibilities with a partner, spouse, or significant other), their likelihood of success is increased (Wilbur et al., 2003). Specific activities should be designed to encourage participants to have discussions with their partners or spouses about sharing responsibilities. This will enable them to exercise without worrying about other household tasks. If household responsibilities are shared, people are more likely to take time to participate in health-enhancing levels of physical activity.

▪ *Provide follow-up.* Program leaders should check in with participants periodically throughout the intervention—either with phone calls or home visits—to answer questions, provide encouragement, and remind them to complete activity logs (see figure 9.1; Robertson et al., 2001; Wilbur et al.,

Directions

Please date and fill in the exercise logs as you complete the exercises. At the end of the fourth week, tear out the completed log sheets and mail them to us using the attached envelope. The final four log sheets can simply be brought in to your last testing session. We will be contacting you to arrange a testing date.

Exercise Log Week 1   Date _____

Session 1   Repetitions

	Set 1	Set 2	Set 3	Band color
Chair stand	_____	_____	_____	_____
Heel raise	_____	_____	_____	_____
Chest press	_____	_____	_____	_____
Shoulder press	_____	_____	_____	_____
Triceps kickback	_____	_____	_____	_____
Hammer curl	_____	_____	_____	_____
Hip abduction	_____	_____	_____	_____

	Trial 1	Trial 2	Trial 3	
Tiptoes	_____	_____	_____	Check after completed
Tight rope walker	_____	_____	_____	
Yoga stork	_____	_____	_____	
Slide trombone	_____	_____	_____	

Session 2   Repetitions

	Set 1	Set 2	Set 3	Band color
Chair stand	_____	_____	_____	_____
Heel raise	_____	_____	_____	_____
Chest press	_____	_____	_____	_____
Shoulder press	_____	_____	_____	_____
Triceps kickback	_____	_____	_____	_____
Hammer curl	_____	_____	_____	_____
Hip abduction	_____	_____	_____	_____

	Trial 1	Trial 2	Trial 3	
Tiptoes	_____	_____	_____	Check after completed
Tight rope walker	_____	_____	_____	
Yoga stork	_____	_____	_____	
Slide trombone	_____	_____	_____	

FIGURE 9.1 Sample log for home-based participants to track their exercise program participation.

From L. Ransdell, M. Dinger, J. Huberty, and K. Miller, 2009, *Developing Effective Physical Activity Programs* (Champaign, IL: Human Kinetics). Reprinted from *DAMET News*, University of Utah Department of Exercise and Sport Science.

2003). Ideally, a postintervention follow-up should occur several months after the participant has completed the intervention. Programs that include follow-up—preferably during and after an intervention—are typically more successful than those that simply tell participants what to do at the pretesting stage of the program.

▪ *Provide low-cost activities that can be completed at home.* Activity leaders should develop activities that are low cost and easy to perform at home (e.g., strength activities using body weight, stretch bands, soup cans, plastic bottles filled with water, physio balls, or dumbbells) (Robertson et al., 2001). People are more likely to participate in activities over the long term if the activities can be done at home for minimal cost using materials supplied by program administrators.

Barriers to Home-Based Physical Activity Programs

Even though home-based physical activity programs are among the most convenient and cost-effective programs available, people in this setting also experience barriers. Knowledge of barriers to home-based programming and potential ways to overcome these barriers can significantly increase the success of a program. Following are some established barriers to participating in home-based physical activity programs and suggested solutions for overcoming them.

▪ *Time to develop programs is significant.* Anyone who is challenged to develop a home-based physical activity program should realize that the time required up front to develop materials such as Web sites, videotapes, DVDs, or CDs is extensive. To minimize this barrier, program designers should develop programs that are simple and drawn from other, previously developed materials where possible. They should also pilot test their programs to discover any problems or shortcomings. Consulting with people from a variety of backgrounds is advisable so one person is not expected to design and act in the video, DVD, or CD and develop the Web site. Tapping the expertise of people from a variety of areas undoubtedly improves the quality and effectiveness of a program.

▪ *Those who need home-based programs may have low adherence rates.* Interestingly, people who need physical activity programs the most (e.g., the frail elderly, less fit people, those with illness or injury, those taking more than one prescription drug) are less likely to adhere to program requirements (Robertson et al., 2001). To minimize this barrier, designers should promote the significant benefits of a physical activity program and make the program progressive (so as not to cause injury), evidence-based, and supported with personnel available via phone calls or e-mails.

▪ *Lack of social connectivity can hinder home-based programs.* Because home-based groups don't meet regularly for exercise, some people perceive a lack of social connectivity—which can interfere with the motivation to participate. Carmeli and colleagues (2006) studied participants recovering from hip replacement surgery. These people, whether they were in a home-based or class-based program, similarly improved their physical functioning. Interestingly, participants in the class-based program were more likely than those in the home-based program to report positive improvements in vitality, social well-being, and emotional status. To increase the social aspect of a home-based program, participants should be able to access a Web site with a chat room and bulletin board to discuss relevant issues and ask questions of those administering the program. Participants should also be able to contact program administrators via phone or e-mail when important questions arise.

■ *Failure to focus on intrinsic motivation can hinder program success.* For maximum success, participants in home-based programs should be highly motivated. Motivation can be either extrinsic (e.g., medals, certificates, group recognition) or intrinsic (e.g., internal satisfaction felt with accomplishing a goal). Although extrinsic motivation may help a person get started in a home-based program, intrinsic motivation is what will help them continue. Those with lower levels of motivation or those who participate in exercise or activity for the social interaction benefits may be less successful with a home-based program. To enhance motivation with home-based programs, program leaders should provide newsletters with program highlights (see figure 9.2) and progress reports. Participants should be asked regularly about their level of motivation, and if it is lacking, program leaders should find ways to facilitate motivation at an individual level.

■ *Lack of creativity and variety can hinder program success.* Because of the cost involved, home-based programs are limited to calisthenics or exercises using body weight, dumbbells, or stretch bands. Other types of equipment and activities, although desirable for maintaining the interest of those participating, are not readily available for home-based activities. To prevent boredom due to a lack of variety in the activities, program leaders should demonstrate new exercises regularly, give away new or different equipment throughout the program, and have contests to see who can break various records.

Figure 9.3 illustrates a page from a home-based exercise manual designed for seniors (e.g., pictures of exercises) that includes simple exercises that do not require too much specialty equipment.

Sample Successful Home-Based Physical Activity Programs

In the sections that follow, several examples of home-based physical activity programs are presented. These programs are typically low-cost, creative, and effective ways to increase physical activity in a population that is sometimes resistant to activity.

Volume 1, Issue 1

May 2001

DAMET News

University of Utah Department of Exercise and Sport Science

DAMET Leaders Battling "Post-Intervention Depression"

Just kidding!! We thought that headline would get your attention. Seriously though, we are missing everyone! I'm filling in for Darcie, Alison, and Jenny—all of whom are taking well-deserved breaks after a tough semester of work.

Alison is heading South (to Tennessee and North Carolina) to work on her golf game and tan. She is also writing lesson plans for her work with the National Youth Sports Program (NYSP) this summer. That program, which starts mid-June, is funded by the NCAA and it targets underserved youth to help them increase their physical activity and learn some valuable life skills.

Darcie is heading to South Dakota to spend the summer with her boyfriend (fiancee'?) ! I'm wondering if we'll ever see her again!

Jenny, who collected the Dept. of Exercise and Sport Science "Outstanding ESS Graduate" award, has finished the MCAT and is planning to relax a bit this summer.

Lynda just bought a new mountain bike (Cannondale, Full Suspension V2000) and is planning to take it on the trails as much as possible this summer!

We'd love to hear updates on your athletic endeavors during the summer so PLEASE make sure and write us with occasional updates on things. It is so much fun to hear from everyone—I'm sure the entire group would love to hear

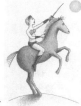

DAMET Women Strive to Continue Their Physical Activity After 12 weeks with Dr. R., Alison, Darcie and Jenny

what you're up to!!

Remember that the DAMET Picnic will be held on Thursday, May 24th at 6pm. More details will follow via email.

Special points of interest:

- May Sport and Recreation Events
- DAMET Leaders Battling "Post-Intervention Depression"
- Does Exercise Reduce the Risk of Breast Cancer?
- Exercise and Adolescent Girls
- Exercise and Social Influences

Inside this issue:

Does Physical Activity Reduce Risk of Breast Cancer?

Does physical activity reduce the risk of breast cancer? Theoretically, it might because exercise can lower levels of female reproductive hormones—which, in excess, may be related to breast cancer. Additionally, physical activity can help women boost their immune system and maintain a lower body weight.

Results of epidemiologic studies seeking the answer to this question are inconsistent. Some studies maintain that risk is reduced in more active women, while others maintain that risk is increased. This study prospectively examined the relationship between physical activity and breast cancer in a cohort of over 39,000 women who were 45 years or older. Results indicated that physical activity was not *uniformly* associated with decreased breast cancer risk. However, when postmenopausal women were examined separately, the most active group experienced a statistically non-significant 24% decrease in risk when compared to the least active group.

Lee, I.M., Rexrode, K.M., Cook, N.R., Hennekens, C.H., & Buring, J.E. (2001). Physical activity and breast cancer risk: The Women's Health Study (United States). Cancer Causes and Control, 12, 137-145.

FIGURE 9.2 Sample newsletter used to help motivate participants from a home-based exercise program, Daughters and Mothers Exercising Together (DAMET).

Reprinted from *DAMET News*, University of Utah Department of Exercise and Sport Science.

Home-Based Activity Program (HBAP)

Taggart, Taggart, and Siedentop (1986) described a 12-week physical activity program for elementary school–aged children with poor fitness levels and low-level motor skills. In this (somewhat older) study, physical education

Exercise Descriptions From a Home-Based Senior Fitness Program

Chest Press
Wrap the band around the middle of the back and then grasp the ends of the band next to the armpits. Press the arms straight out, keeping the shoulders down. Slowly return to the starting position.

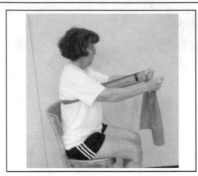

Shoulder Press
Begin this exercise while sitting on the center of the exercise band. Hold an end of the band in each hand at shoulder height with your arms bent. Press the hands upward until the arms are fully extended and return slowly to the starting position

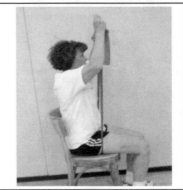

Triceps Kick Back
Begin in a sitting position with the center of the band under both feet. Hold the ends of the band with the elbows flexed. Press right forearm backward until the elbow is straight, and then return slowly to the starting position. Repeat for the left arm.

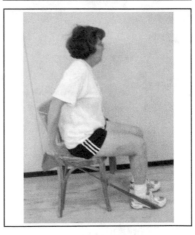

FIGURE 9.3 **This page provides an example of a home-based exercise program for seniors.**
© Terry-Ann Spitzer Gibson.

teachers (called "parenters") developed "fitness homework" and collaborated with parents to improve fitness levels and motor coordination in children (*n* = 12) who failed to attain health-related fitness criteria in three or more areas (e.g., cardiorespiratory endurance, abdominal strength, lower back strength, shoulder girdle strength, lower back and hip flexibility, and body composition). Physical education teachers trained parents to implement family contracting, monitor physical activity during nonschool hours, and administer fitness tests to check progress. As a result of this program, participation in physical activity (time in minutes) increased 49% from pre- to postintervention. Health-related fitness also increased across most of the measured variables. Although this study had several limitations (e.g., small sample size, no control group), it is worth mentioning because the methods used to facilitate change in physical activity in children were unique.

Moving Forward

Moving Forward was a randomized controlled trial that compared the effectiveness of a 12-week home-based program to a contact control group in terms of facilitating changes in physical activity, fitness, vigor, fatigue, and motivational readiness in women (n = 86) recovering from breast cancer treatment (Pinto et al., 2005). Women in the home-based program were tested on their stage of change and received tailored face-to-face instruction about exercising, monitoring their heart rate, using activity logs, and wearing pedometers. Throughout the intervention, women were phoned to monitor physical activity participation, identify problems, solve barriers, and reinforce efforts.

The contact control group received cancer survivor tip sheets, and they were asked not to change their current level of physical activity. They received weekly phone calls from program officials and were asked about their posttreatment symptoms. Compared to women in the contact control group, women in the home-based program reported significantly more minutes of total physical activity and moderate to vigorous activity, better fitness test results, more vigor, and less fatigue. Psychosocial variables measured did not change, possibly because there was no support group with whom to discuss postcancer treatment issues.

Preoperative Preparation

Keays and colleagues (2006) studied two groups of 12 matched patients with anterior cruciate ligament deficiency (ACLD) who were awaiting surgery. ACLD patients were asked to participate in a 6-week preoperative home-based program or serve in a control group. Twelve matched uninjured controls were also included in the study for "normal" comparative information. The intervention group was trained by physiotherapists on how to do seven open and closed kinetic chain exercises designed to strengthen hamstrings, quadriceps, and calves; stretching, plyometrics, and balance activities were also included. Members of the intervention group were asked to participate in the exercise program daily for 30 minutes and track their participation. Members of the control and normal groups continued with their usual activity. Participants in the study were measured pre- and postintervention on knee stability, muscle strength, standing balance, and functional performance on tests of agility and hopping.

Compared to those in the other two groups, participants in the preoperative intervention program increased their quad strength and improved their single-leg balance and agility significantly more than those in the control group. This ability to successfully use a home-based preoperative intervention to improve strength, balance, and agility in those with ACLD has significant implications for ACL surgery preparation and recovery.

A variety of home-based programs are available. Several have been covered in previous chapters (e.g., chapter 4 on women, and chapter 6 on older adults) because those populations tend to respond favorably to home-based interventions. Therefore, in an effort to show the breadth of home-based programming available, the programs covered in this section were designed to address children's physical activity after school, preoperative preparation, and breast cancer treatment.

GETTING STARTED

Checklist for Developing Successful Home-Based Programs

❑ Develop preprogram training sessions to inform participants of program expectations.

❑ Plan on spending a lot of time developing the program (versus implementing it).

❑ Provide a high level of detail in a simple and easy-to-use format so participants can easily follow the program.

❑ Expect a reasonable time commitment (e.g., 30 to 60 minutes per exercise session).

❑ Teach participants how to negotiate role balance with their families.

❑ Provide follow-up contacts with participants.

❑ Make programs low in cost and high in convenience.

❑ Find ways to increase social connectivity—even if participants will be exercising separately.

❑ Be prepared to deal with low motivation; participants may struggle without positive influences and interactions with others.

Family-Based Physical Activity Programs

Families, including spouses, significant others, parents, and children, are powerful change agents. They can influence many lifestyle choices including physical activity and dietary habits (Aarnio, Winter, Kujala, & Kaprio, 1997;

Beunen & Thomis, 1999; Fogelholm, Nuutinen, Pasanen, Myohanen, & Saatela, 1999; Wrotniak, Epstein, Paluch, & Roemmich, 2005). Family-based physical activity programs target at least two related people who live in the same household, although programs targeting multiple generations of families exist (Ransdell, Robertson, Ornes, & Moyer-Mileur, 2004).

Most of the early family-based programs were designed to strengthen families to prevent substance abuse or minimize its impact on a family. The main activities of these programs included facilitating family bonding and improving conflict resolution (described in Redmond, Spoth, Shin, & Lepper, 1999). Family-based programs to lower risk of heart disease have also been developed (Higgins, 2000). Two of the better-known family-based programs designed to address heart health include the Tromso Family Study (Knutsen

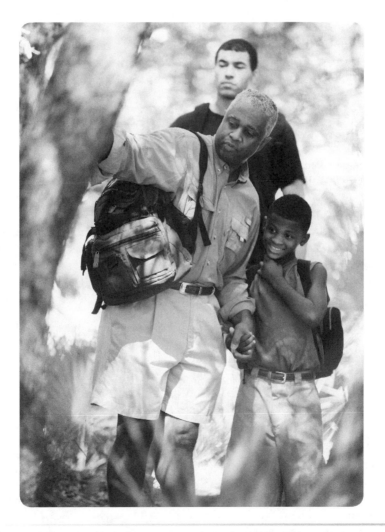

Families that participate in physical activity together gain significant benefits in terms of bonding, improving health and fitness, and developing lifelong patterns of physical activity.

& Knutsen, 1991), which targeted men with CHD and their families, and the British Family Heart Study (Pyke, Wood, Kinmonth, & Thompson, 1997), which sought to change unhealthy lifestyle behaviors in middle-aged couples. Programs that proactively encourage families to increase physical activity to prevent hypokinetic disease have only recently emerged (Ransdell et al., 2004; Rodearmel et al., 2006; Rodearmel et al., 2007). Because families spend so much time together, the family environment is very important for acquiring and maintaining physical activity behaviors (Wrotniak et al., 2005). The paragraphs that follow describe several factors related to the success of family-based programs.

Factors Related to Successful Family-Based Physical Activity Programs

Given the important role that families play in determining behavior, program planners should understand the factors related to the success of a family-based physical activity program. Following are some things program planners can do to positively influence physical activity at the familial level:

■ *Encourage families to model active behavior.* Physical activity is modeled by families (Ritchie, Welk, Styne, Gerstein, & Crawford, 2005). Because studies have shown that parental modeling is highly related to physical activity behaviors in children (Richie et al., 2005; Wrotniak et al., 2005), it is important that family-based interventions build in modeling opportunities for parents. Family members reinforce typical behaviors, and they discourage unique behaviors. For example, if a mother decides to work out at 6 p.m. instead of cooking dinner and serving it to the family (which is her usual behavior for that time of day), the family may not be supportive of this change in routine. To the contrary, if family members enjoy playing tennis together, it is highly likely that they will play tennis together as a family activity—even if it is at 6 p.m., the usual dinner time.

■ *Make interventions low cost.* Families with children sometimes struggle to make ends meet. Families struggling to put food on the table have to make difficult decisions about budgetary cuts. Given the importance of providing low-cost services to families, a physical activity intervention targeting families should be low in cost and high in benefits. The good news is that family interventions reach out to multiple members of a family; therefore, they should be more cost-effective than individual interventions (Bonomi, Boudreau, Fishman, Meenan, & Revicki, 2005).

■ *Consider using the family systems theory.* The family systems theory maintains that the family is an organized hierarchy of subsystems that influence each other (Bonomi et al., 2005). Several factors, including degree of cohesion, adaptability to change, communication, and mutual agreement and understanding, can affect the overall well-being of a family and ultimately the success of a family-based program. Therefore, successful programs should be designed to increase cohesion and improve communication. Some of the more successful interventions were designed to help families get to know each other better by teaching communication and conflict resolution skills (Ransdell et al., 2004; Teufel-Shone, Drummond, & Rawiel, 2005; Wrotniak et al., 2005). For example, Pollner and Stein (1996, as cited in Flora & Faulkner, 2006) described the use of "narrative maps" whereby people, practices, and problems encountered are discussed in the context of various age groups. These narrative maps are powerful because they can decrease anxiety, increase motivation, and improve morale in parents and their children. In general, these discussions can change perceptions about generational differences and move family members toward common ground (Flora & Faulkner, 2006).

■ *Encourage families to replace media use with physical activity.* Electronic media, including television, video games, computers, portable music devices, and other electronic devices, are omnipresent in today's society. Several researchers have determined that heavy media use is related to decreased physical activity and increased obesity, especially in youth (Bagley, Salmon, & Crawford, 2006; Bar-Or et al., 1998; Clocksin, Watson, & Ransdell, 2002; Salmon, Timperio, Telford, Carver, & Crawford, 2005). In addition, as families are increasingly using media, they are interacting with each other less. Limiting electronic media use will "force" face-to-face communication and hopefully increase interactions between human beings (Ritchie et al., 2005). Physical activity can be increased with additional attention to facilitating face-to-face interactions and substituting electronic media use with physical activity.

■ *Teach parents how to create a healthy home environment.* Intervention specialists should teach parents how to create a healthy home environment using techniques such as reinforcement, stimulus control, and environmental restructuring (Wrotniak et al., 2005). For example, if a family is working on environmental restructuring, parents can install a basketball hoop in the driveway for children who like to play basketball or purchase hockey nets for children who like to play street or roller hockey. They can also remove televisions from children's bedrooms or limit TV, computer, or video game use to limit sedentary leisure-time activity opportunities and increase active leisure pursuits. It is also important for parents trying to increase physical activity for their children to provide support in the form of information and equipment, and to provide emotional support such as encouragement and a positive attitude (Bagley et al., 2006).

Barriers to Family-Based Physical Activity Programs

Contact with the family occurs frequently. Given that families interact so much with each other and that family habits are hard to change, it is likely that barriers to family-based physical activity programs exist. Knowledge of these barriers can make the difference between a successful and unsuccessful program. Following is a list of some barriers to family-based programming—and some ways to overcome them.

▪ *Few programs have been developed and tested.* One of the largest barriers to developing successful family-based physical activity programs is that very few programs have been developed and tested—especially compared to other types of physical activity interventions. As more programs become available, dissemination will increase and families will have more opportunities to participate in activity together and learn additional strategies for increasing physical activity behavior.

▪ *Some families prefer to participate in more sedentary activities.* Physical activity can be difficult in that it requires participants to work hard, increase their heart rate, and even sweat. Therefore, another barrier to increasing physical activity is that some families prefer more sedentary activities (e.g., reading, watching TV, using the computer). Changing household patterns to emphasize physical activity rather than sedentary activity is a challenge (Salmon et al., 2005). The first step toward overcoming the preference for more sedentary activities is to substitute sedentary behaviors with more active behaviors. For example, rather than reading a book while sitting, family members can take turns reading books to each other while other family members skip rope or use exercise equipment. Family members can also incorporate physical activity into watching TV. If a game show is on, family members can guess the answers to questions. Those who get answers correct can tell other members of the family which physical activity they have to do (e.g., 5 push-ups or 20 sit-ups). If a favorite TV show is on, family members can each choose a character on the show and every time their character appears, they have to do a specific type or amount of physical activity.

▪ *Family schedules are typically very busy.* A third barrier to family-based interventions is that finding time in family schedules these days is difficult. The most common reason for dropping out of family-based physical activity programs is a lack of time. Families are often going from dusk till dawn with a variety of commitments, including academic expectations, job-related requirements, and extracurricular activities. Therefore, it is very important to provide families with choices for physical activity programming. Family-based physical activity programming should be designed to meet the needs of a variety of family structures.

Sample Successful Family-Based Physical Activity Programs

The sections that follow provide some examples of successful family-based physical activity programs. These programs provide examples for modeling active behavior, replacing media use with activity, and training parents to create a supportive home environment.

America on the Move

Rodearmel and colleagues (2006, 2007) published two papers describing family-based programs designed to increase physical activity and positively affect dietary habits. In the first study (Rodearmel et al., 2006), 105 families with at least one child (8 to 12 years old) at risk for overweight were assigned to a 13-week intervention (INT) or control (CTL) group. Both groups received pedometers and step and dietary logs, and baseline and postintervention data were collected. Family members were asked to compile data on a refrigerator magnet, which was mailed back to the researchers after weeks 3 and 10. Those in the INT group were instructed to increase their physical activity by taking 2,000 or more steps per day and consume two servings per day of cereal (one for breakfast and one as a snack) because cereal is lower in calories and higher in nutrient density than many of the breakfast and snack foods available today. The overall goal for the INT group was to decrease caloric intake or increase caloric expenditure by 100 calories per day. Those in the CTL group were told to maintain their usual pattern of activity and diet. At the end of 13 weeks, compared to the CTL group, the INT group walked more (steps per day) and ate more cereal (cups per day), and there was a positive and statistically significant impact on BMI for age in children and BMI and percent body fat in their parents. Interestingly, the effects of this first intervention were seen more in girls and their mothers than in boys and their fathers.

In the second version of this study (Rodearmel et al., 2007), 192 families were randomly assigned to a 6-month intervention group (INT) or a self-monitor group (SM). Families from both groups met with study staff on six occasions (e.g., at enrollment, after a 2-week baseline, and at the end of weeks 6, 12, 18, and 24) so the staff could collect data, ask questions, and encourage continuation in the study. Both groups were asked to record their data on refrigerator magnets and use reminder stickers on the bathroom mirror. The INT group was similar to that in the previous study in that participants were told to walk an additional 2,000 steps per day and eliminate 100 calories per day from their diets (e.g., replace sugar with a noncaloric sweetener such as sucralose). They were also taught about label reading, baking with sucralose, the benefits of eating breakfast, eating and preparing meals at home, and eating five fruits or vegetables per day. The SM group used pedometers and recorded their physical activity on logs, but they were not given instructions to increase physical activity or change their diet until the end of the study. During the 6-month program, only 16% of the sample dropped out. Children in the INT group didn't meet their step goals, but they did report a significant increase in steps per day compared to the SM children. Children in the INT group also reported eating fewer sugar-sweetened desserts compared to their counterparts in the SM group. Overall, both groups of children decreased their BMI for age; however, the INT group had a higher percentage of children who maintained or reduced their BMI for age compared to the SM group.

Parents from both groups maintained their weight and BMI throughout the 6-month program.

Family Fitness

Hopper, Munoz, Gruber, and Nguyen (2005) compared the effectiveness of a 20-week school- and home-based physical activity and nutrition program to a traditional program in third-grade children from six area elementary schools. Children (n = 238) were divided into intervention (INT) and control (CTL) groups. Those in the INT group received a health-related fitness school-based program plus a home-based program whereby parents and their children completed various worksheets, homework, and activities related to behavior change in exchange for points. Because the program was based on social learning theory, parents were asked to practice role modeling, behavior rehearsal, goal setting, behavioral cueing, and reinforcement of desired behaviors. The CTL group participated in traditional physical education classes three times a week for 30 minutes each and nutrition education classes twice a week for 30 minutes. Compared to participants in the CTL group, those in the INT group scored higher on exercise and nutrition knowledge tests. Additionally, those in the INT group showed greater reductions in fat intake compared to those in the CTL group. No differences or changes in physical measures such as percent body fat and cholesterol were reported.

This program is unique in that parents were asked to work with their children outside the traditional school programs to change behaviors. Although parental changes were not measured, this program was modestly effective in changing knowledge and dietary behaviors in children.

La Diabetes Y La Union Familiar (Diabetes and the Family)

Teufel-Shone and colleagues (2005) developed a physical activity and nutrition program designed to build family support for Hispanic patients with diabetes. The program was the result of collaboration between a university and two community health agencies. Because the Hispanic culture places strong emphasis on family connectedness, intervention developers believed that this setting would be ideal for intervening with high-risk Hispanic diabetics and their families. In this study, *promotoras* (or community leaders who promote health) were trained to teach families (n = 72 subjects and 177 supportive family members) educational content and lead activities designed to increase knowledge about diabetes risk factors, and improve self-confidence to change dietary and physical activity behaviors.

Over a 12-week period, there were 10 contacts including 3 home visits, 5 educational sessions, and 2 celebratory events. The program, based on social learning theory, was designed to teach families team building and communication skills, and build and reinforce family-wide self-esteem and confidence in the ability to change dietary and physical activity behaviors. During home visits, promotoras worked with families to collectively set goals, discuss overcoming barriers to changing diet and physical activity habits, and develop plans to sustain behavior change.

As a result of this program, participants significantly decreased their intake of sweet (noncarbonated) drinks and increased physical activity within their families. Changes in family support, including communication and cohesive behaviors, were not statistically significant, although they were mentioned frequently during postintervention interviews with participants. Interestingly, changes were more likely to occur in females within the family than in males. Although this program did not have a comparison control group, it demonstrated significant changes in dietary and physical activity behaviors thought to contribute to diabetes risk. It is worthwhile to continue examining these types of interventions because they meet a need within a community that is often devastated by diabetes.

Checklist for Developing Successful Physical Activity Programs With Families

❑ Encourage parents to model physically active lifestyles.

❑ Offer programs at a low cost—given the typical expenses of a family.

❑ Include family systems theory, which encourages increased cohesion, improved communication, and conflict resolution strategies.

❑ Whenever possible, replace media use with physical activity.

❑ Train parents to create a supportive and active home environment.

GETTING STARTED

Church-Based Physical Activity Programs

Church-based programs are efforts led by a church community to improve the health of members through education, screening, referral, treatment, and group support (Ransdell & Rehling, 1996). Churches are unique and logical settings in which to develop physical activity programs because they have (a) physical resources (e.g., large meeting facilities), (b) a mission that promotes mental and physical health, (c) spiritual influences that are not typically available from other community entities, (d) groups of volunteers who value philanthropy, (e) media access, (f) strong social networking, and (g) the ability to reach people from a variety of social and economic backgrounds (Ransdell & Rehling, 1996). To date, church-based programs have been used most frequently and most successfully with older adults and African American populations, probably because these two populations comprise the majority of churchgoers in the United States (Ransdell & Rehling, 1996). The next section describes factors related to success with church-based physical activity programs.

LIVERPOOL JOHN MOORES UNIVERSITY
LEARNING SERVICES

Factors Related to Successful Church-Based Physical Activity Programs

Peterson, Atwood, and Yates (2002) and Ransdell and Rehling (1996) described the following recommendations to ensure success with church-based physical activity programs.

■ *Form community partnerships.* To save money, take advantage of accessible expertise, and avoid duplication of services, partnerships should be sought with existing community entities (e.g., YMCAs, local colleges and universities, health clubs, school physical education programs). A wonderful example of an effective partnership is Fitness through Churches funded by the American Heart Association, initiated by the University of North Carolina, and delivered in churches throughout North Carolina (Hatch et al., 1986, as cited in Peterson et al., 2002).

■ *Build on the church mission of serving and caring for others.* Churches are valued within communities for their guidance relative to spiritual, physical, and mental health. They also provide a significant source of social support, which can help facilitate behavior change.

■ *Encourage church leaders to support programs.* The most successful church-based programs have garnered significant and sustained participation by pastors, church boards, and volunteers. When those individuals or groups are involved, the congregation is more likely to buy into the program.

■ *Form a wellness ministry.* A wellness ministry, consisting of church leaders, members, and others with expertise in wellness should be formed so programs can be planned and workloads can be delegated. Sharing workloads for organizing these programs should help prevent the burnout that sometimes occurs with church volunteers.

Barriers to Church-Based Physical Activity Programs

Despite the fact that many church-based programs have reported high levels of success, these programs still have barriers. Lasater, Wells, Carleton, and Elder (1986) surveyed church personnel and reported several common barriers to implementing church-based programs. Following is a list of several of those barriers and solutions for overcoming them.

■ *Significant time commitment.* Volunteers in churches tend to contribute a lot of their own time. Because of the gradual decline in the number of volunteers at churches and the increased responsibilities for those who do volunteer, burnout and stress-related conditions are significant concerns (Wells, DePue, Lasater, & Carleton, 1988). Given this risk of burnout, volunteers may not agree to work on a project if they perceive that it will take too much time. To minimize the time commitment of a new physical activity program, church leaders should recruit as many volunteers as possible to share the workload, and they should offer continual training, support, and recognition to those who deliver programs (Bopp et al., 2007). Churches should also partner with other community organizations that have similar goals for increasing physical activity in the community, and consider using existing curricula for a program so they do not have to reinvent the wheel. Because church patrons need a reason to invest time in a new program, church leaders can be highly influential in promoting the program.

▪ *Facility scheduling.* Churches are busy places. Because they serve a number of entities within a community, facility scheduling can be challenging. Additionally, church leaders may be hesitant to add a new program for fear that it will take away volunteers or participants from an existing program. To overcome these barriers, church leaders should seek out other facilities (if necessary) or figure out ways to creatively schedule events (e.g., alternate programs or split facilities in half to maximize space usage).

▪ *Lack of information about successful programs.* A final barrier to delivering successful church-based programs is that most programs have not been studied using experimental, randomized, and controlled designs (Peterson et al., 2002). Therefore, it is difficult to ascertain which factors are most relevant to facilitating behavior change, and it is difficult to conclude that any behavior change resulted from the intervention (and not other factors). Additionally, the dissemination of information about successful church-based health promotion programs has been fragmented. If information about successful programs were disseminated more systematically and thoroughly, it is possible that money could be saved because successful programs could be used by congregations that do not have the money to recreate programs from scratch.

Sample Successful Church-Based Physical Activity Programs

The successful church-based physical activity programs described in this section serve as models for effective programming in a church-based setting.

Aerobic Fitness and Stretch N Health Programs

Rohm-Young & Stewart (2006) compared the effectiveness of a 6-month church-based Stretch N Health (SH) program to an aerobic fitness program (AF) in African American women (n = 196 from 11 churches in the Baltimore area). Focus groups were used to plan the interventions. Participants in both programs received comparable health information including an individualized physical activity plan and education about health-related fitness status as assessed during baseline testing. The physical activity plan included recommendations for building up to 30 minutes of moderate-intensity activity five times per week.

Participants in the AF group had the opportunity to attend a weekly 1-hour class for a period of 6 months. Physical activity and educational materials were included in the sessions. Women were asked to pray for each other as they adopted the exercise program, and they were paired with another participant who provided social support and encouragement. Participants in the SH program were offered weekly low-intensity stretching classes and health lectures on topics of their choice. Classes for both the SH and AF groups were held at participating churches at convenient times, and they were led by certified fitness instructors from the African American community.

Attendance at SH and AF classes was low (24%), and neither group increased its energy expenditure significantly. SH and AF groups were successful in reducing sedentary behavior from baseline (26% and 18% decline, respectively), and those with higher social support and physical functioning scores at baseline were more likely to increase their participation in physical activity, regardless of group assignment. Researchers concluded that the churches were simply sites in which to conduct the intervention—rather than true partners. In addition, many women in the study were obese, yet generally without cardiovascular or other hypokinetic diseases. Those who attended the program did experience improvements in physical activity behavior, health-related fitness, and psychological health.

Faith on the Move

Faith on the Move was a culturally tailored, randomized trial comparing a faith-based (FB) program to a culturally tailored (CT) program for African American women (n = 59) (Fitzgibbon et al., 2005). The goal of the 12-week program, based on social cognitive theory, was to test the efficacy of both programs in terms of weight loss, dietary fat consumption, and physical activity. Program sessions for both groups were delivered twice weekly for 45 to 90 minutes (e.g., sometimes 45 minutes of education and interaction was combined with 45 minutes of exercise; other times, participants exercised for 45 to 60 minutes). Session topics included the use of daily self-monitoring of physical activity and food intake, reinforcement, modeling, stimulus control, and social support. Women in the FB group received scripture readings in addition to information about exercise and nutrition topics. Attendance was comparable in both groups (i.e., approximately 51% of women in both groups attended ≥75% of the sessions), and women from FB and CT groups lost weight (2.6 and 1.6 kg, respectively). Total energy expenditure (physical activity) increased significantly in the CT group but not the FB group.

Health-e-AME

Wilcox and colleagues (2007) designed a large-scale church-based physical activity program for African Methodist Episcopal churches in South Carolina. Using the "train-the-trainer" model, 889 congregants from 303 churches were trained to deliver three programs, based on the social ecological and transtheoretical models. *Praise aerobics* incorporated light, moderate, and vigorous physical activity set to familiar gospel music. *Chair exercises*, also set to gospel music, were used with people who had medical restrictions that precluded walking. *Walking*, the preferred activity for many adults, was designed to reach the majority of churchgoers. Spiritual and religious messages were integrated throughout the three physical activity programs, and behavior change skills were taught during the first several weeks of the program. The Health-e-AME program has a Web site to guide instructors and participants. Topics on the Web site include general information about physical activity, resource links, a list of participating churches, photos of training events, and copies of training materials.

Although results of this program are forthcoming, preliminary evaluations using the RE-AIM framework (reach, effectiveness, adoption, implementation, and maintenance) were conducted via telephone with a random sample of church health program directors. (Information about the RE-AIM framework can be found at www.re-aim.org.) During the first year of offering the program, 80% of churches had at least one program; by the second year, only 54% of the churches reported implementing at least one physical activity program. The most common problems were poor attendance and a lack of responsiveness to these programs (Bopp et al., 2007). Middle-aged African American women were the most likely participants in the program, but churches had difficulties continuing to offer physical activity sessions because of the lack of interest (Bopp et al., 2007). The unique aspects of this program include the community partnerships formed (e.g., university and church), the theoretical foundations of the program (e.g., social ecological and transtheoretical model), the involvement of church pastors, and unanticipated increases in the physical activity behaviors of the trainers.

Checklist for Developing Successful Programs in Churches

❏ Form partnerships with other community entities with common goals and interests.

❏ Build on the church mission of serving and caring for others.

❏ Encourage church leaders to support and promote programs.

❏ Form a wellness ministry.

❏ As much as possible, minimize the time commitment of volunteers and participants (i.e., share responsibilities, make the program fun and interesting).

GETTING STARTED

Medical Community-Based Physical Activity Programs

Physical activity programs based in the medical community and delivered by doctors, nurses, or other medical personnel have the potential to be very successful because of the high regard with which the medical community is held. Amani-Golshani (2006) reported that over 80% of patients agreed or strongly agreed that they would exercise if a doctor advised it. Therefore, physical activity programs administered in a medical setting are an important strategy to consider for reaching increasingly inactive populations. Physical activity programs supported by the medical community are designed to teach medical personnel to conduct brief activity counseling, distribute print materials, and administer follow-up phone calls to patients (Eakin, Brown, Marshall, Mummery, & Larsen, 2004). Such programs have reported significant success in helping patients change short-term physical activity behavior; however, long-term success is still being examined (Eakin et al., 2004).

Factors Related to Successful Medical Community-Based Physical Activity Programs

Medical community–based interventions provide a unique opportunity to facilitate change in a population that is often inactive: patients with various health problems. This section delineates factors related to successful medical community physical activity programs as described by Douglas, Torrance, van Teijlingen, Meloni, & Kerr (2006) and Taylor (2003).

▪ *Consider predisposing, reinforcing, and enabling characteristics.* The first factor that can increase success in a medical setting is to consider the predisposing, reinforcing, and enabling characteristics of the target population (Taylor, 2003). For example, medical professionals should be aware of *predisposing* factors such as attributes and characteristics of patients prior to recommending physical activity programming. *Reinforcing* factors, or resources, supportive policies, or services that patients can access are also important to consider in the process. Finally, *enabling* factors, or social support or praise, should be considered prior to advising patients on physical activity behaviors.

▪ *Recommend walking.* Walking is the most popular physical activity in the world. It is convenient, it can be done with friends in almost any setting, and minimal equipment is needed. As long as mobility is not an issue, walking is the activity in which people are most likely to participate.

▪ *Train medical personnel to conduct counseling.* Medical personnel may or may not have confidence and training to counsel people relative to increasing their level of physical activity in a safe and reasonable fashion. For this reason, medical personnel should be trained, preferably by someone with expertise in exercise science, exercise psychology, or physical education, to counsel previously inactive people. Because this is not an easy job, those who do this should be well trained so they are confident in delivering information.

▪ *Make PA counseling as time-efficient and cost-effective as possible.* Physicians' offices are typically very busy. For that reason, those who counsel patients about physical activity should use predeveloped handouts, Web sites, brochures, and other materials. If these materials are available for a low cost, they can be given to patients to reinforce information discussed during counseling.

Barriers to Medical Community-Based Physical Activity Programs

Receiving physical activity advice from someone in the medical community typically results in action. However, barriers to promoting physical activity through the medical community exist. The most commonly cited barriers to promoting physical activity in medical communities—and proposed ways to overcome those barriers—are presented in this section. Bull, Schipper, Jamrozik, and Blanksby (1997); Douglas and colleagues (2006); and Ribera, McKenna, and Riddoch (2006) offer more information on this topic.

▪ *Lack of time and confidence.* Physicians, despite their extensive medical backgrounds, may not be trained specifically to help people increase their current level of physical activity. Additionally, they may not schedule extra time to counsel patients to increase their level of activity. To deal with a lack of time and confidence relative to counseling about physical activity, physicians' offices should use predeveloped counseling modules (as discussed earlier), or they should recommend Web sites designed to help patients increase their current level of activity.

▪ *Lack of financial reimbursement.* Medicine is a costly endeavor. Typically, doctors are paid for their time, including appointments with patients. To cope with the cost of time spent counseling patients about increasing their physical activity, physicians should train their assistants to counsel patients about physical activity, and they should use predeveloped counseling modules or prescription pads with recommendations for physical activity participation. They should also partner with various community groups (e.g., YMCAs or colleges or universities) and refer patients to quality physical activity programs in the area. Finally, those from the medical field should collect data about the impact of medical counseling and use it to lobby the government to reimburse doctors for providing exercise or physical activity prescriptions.

▪ *Perception of poor patient compliance.* Medical professionals may perceive that patients do not follow instructions to increase their level of activity. To overcome that barrier, physical activity promotion specialists should share research papers with medical personnel to show them the difference that counseling patients to increase activity—even a small amount—can make. Some excellent resources that document the effectiveness of medical community-based physical activity programs include Aittasalo, Miilunpalo, Stahl, and

Kukkonen-Harjula (2006); Bull and colleagues (1997); Elley, Kerse, Arroll, and Robinson (2003); Ribera and colleagues (2006); and Rose, Lawton, Elley, Dowell, and Fenton (2007).

Sample Successful Medical Community–Based Physical Activity Programs

The programs presented in this section are models for designing effective programs within the medical community.

10,000 Steps Rockhampton

One of the more successful multifaceted community campaigns to increase physical activity, 10,000 Steps Rockhampton, was initiated in Australia. Details of one arm of this program are covered in chapter 10; however, information specific to working with the medical community will be covered here. The goals of this study were to (a) increase general physicians' awareness of the importance of PA promotion in primary care, (b) train physicians in PA counseling techniques, (c) conduct practice visits and provide PA counseling materials and 10,000 Steps Rockhampton resources to physicians, and (d) promote the use of pedometers by giving physicians pedometers to give to their patients (Eakin et al., 2004).

Specifically, 66 general practitioners from 23 practices received resources for and instruction in brief physical activity counseling, and pedometers to use in conjunction with counseling. An evaluation was conducted using the RE-AIM framework, and data were collected pre- and postintervention using a random digit-dial phone survey conducted with residents of Rockhampton and a comparison community.

The majority (91%) of practices agreed to participate in the training, and 58% of general physicians from those practices were trained. At follow-up, 62% displayed a physical activity promotion poster in their offices, 81% reported using the brochures provided, and 70% gave out pedometers to interested patients. Physicians did not report any increase in the proportion of patients counseled on physical activity (it remained around 30%). However, pre- to postintervention data from Rockhampton residents indicated a 31% increase in PA counseling; in the comparison community, a 16% decrease in PA counseling was reported. It seems likely that some components of the program will be maintained because 81% of the general physicians insisted that they planned to continue using the 10,000 Steps Rockhampton brochure, and 68% said they would continue using pedometers.

Physical Activity Prescription Programme (PAPP)

The PAPP program was administered in Finland in an attempt to increase physical activity counseling among physicians in primary care facilities

(Aittasalo et al., 2006). Physicians were trained in person by peers and trainers using a published training protocol called PREX. Upon completing the training, physicians were given a 10-page users guide with sample physical activity logs and exercise prescription pads for patients. They were asked to assess patients' current PA habits; if inadequate, they were instructed to tell patients to exercise and use goal-setting strategies to facilitate success. Physicians were also asked to monitor patient progress. An attempt was made to convert PREX to an electronic format, but technical problems prevented this from occurring in a timely and efficient manner.

The program was evaluated using the RE-AIM framework, and two noteworthy findings were mentioned. First, the PAPP reached health care professionals effectively (i.e., 34% of health centers were using the PREX program). Second, the program was implemented and initiated by local programs so it could be institutionalized. For example, 3,048 exercise prescriptions were delivered, and the percentage of physicians recommending increased PA to patients increased significantly from the beginning to the end of the project. In addition, the PREX program strengthened physicians' confidence with using PA counseling as a strategy for increasing physical activity.

Women's Lifestyle Study

Rose and colleagues (2007) described an ongoing 2-year randomized controlled trial of physical activity counseling (Women's Lifestyle Study) used in primary health care in New Zealand. This study is a follow-up to the modestly successful Green Prescription program that used verbal and written advice to patients from a health professional, followed by 3 months of phone support from exercise specialists (Elley et al., 2003). The Green Prescription program resulted in significant improvements in physical activity and quality of life among previously sedentary adults (40 to 79 years old) over a yearlong period.

In this newer study, physically inactive women (n = 880; 40 to 74 years old) were randomized to either a lifestyle PA intervention or control group. Nurses delivered physical activity interventions, and women in the intervention group received a "lifestyle script" from a primary care nurse. The script recommends moderate-intensity brisk walking (or the equivalent) at a duration and frequency that is individualized for each participant. The presentation of the lifestyle script is followed by 9 months of phone counseling and a face-to-face visit after 6 months. Control group participants receive "usual care" and are asked to maintain their current behaviors because their health is being followed over the next 2 years. Outcome measures, as yet to be reported, include physical activity and fitness, blood pressure, weight, blood lipids, and quality of life.

Checklist for Developing a Successful Medical Community–Based Program

❏ Know predisposing, reinforcing, and enabling factors of patients prior to recommending physical activity.

❏ Train medical personnel to conduct counseling.

❏ Make counseling as time-efficient and cost-effective as possible.

❏ Use predeveloped modules, Web sites, and other community resources to assist with counseling; don't create a program if one already exists.

❏ Use physical activity prescription pads that can be completed and distributed to patients.

❏ For those who are mobile, recommend walking because it is convenient and popular with people recovering from illness or disease.

Worksite-Based Physical Activity Programs

Worksite physical activity programs sponsor activities in the workplace that are designed to improve the health, or in this case, increase the physical activity behavior, of employees (Addley, McQuillan, & Ruddle, 2001). Workplaces are perhaps the ideal locations in which to address health promotion issues because they provide the following (Addley et al., 2001):

- Access to large numbers of people who are part of a larger social community
- An opportunity for positive health messages to be enhanced by social influences
- The potential to reach people who are not easily reached in other ways
- The possibility of disseminating information about a healthy lifestyle to the family and friends of employees outside the targeted workplace

In addition to the many ethical benefits of worksite-based programs, there are economic benefits. Employee participation in worksite physical activity programs is related to the following (Addley et al., 2001; Wynne & Clarkin, 1992):

- Decreased absenteeism
- Decreased accidents
- Lower rates of litigation
- Increased morale and productivity

Some organizations offer worksite physical activity programming to make their workplace more attractive than others and to invest in the health and well-being of their workforce (Wynne & Clarkin, 1992).

Factors Related to Successful Worksite-Based Physical Activity Programs

To ensure success with worksite physical activity programming, several strategies are recommended. These strategies are drawn from Harden, Peersman, Oliver, Mauthen, & Oakley (1999), who conducted a systematic review of 100 worksite interventions, and Dishman, Oldenburg, O'Neal, and Shephard (1998), who conducted a large meta-analysis to examine which variables had the strongest effects on the success of worksite physical activity programs. Following are descriptions of these strategies.

■ *Secure the support of top-level management.* It is imperative that top management support employee participation in a physical activity or exercise program. If managers do not support programming by encouraging employee participation, supporting these programs verbally and financially, or role modeling participation, programs will not last long. Because of the high-pressure workplace common today, employees will not participate if they are not given permission or encouragement to participate.

■ *Focus on modifiable risk factors.* Worksite programs should target things that can be changed (i.e., modifiable risk factors) such as nutrition and physical activity. Programs that focus on these risk factors (rather than nonmodifiable risk factors such as genetic background) are more likely to succeed and result in significant health-related changes.

■ *Tailor the program to the characteristics and needs of the workforce.* The message of individually tailoring activities has been emphasized throughout this book. Using this strategy within the context of worksite physical activity promotion is strongly recommended. Because people do not respond the same to all programs, using focus groups to plan activities and providing a variety of offerings to meet the needs of various constituents is important to the success of any worksite program.

■ *Use behavior modification strategies.* To ensure the success of a worksite-based physical activity program, program facilitators should use behavior modification strategies such as goal setting, positive self-talk, behavior logs, and rewards. Goal setting and providing rewards for effort help participants focus their efforts, and positive self-talk prevents participants from derailing their efforts at behavior change. As is true when working with most of the populations highlighted in this book, attention to behavior modification strategies can significantly enhance the success of a program.

Barriers to Worksite-Based Physical Activity Programs

Although worksite physical activity programs are appealing for a variety of reasons, there are still barriers to making them successful (Addley et al., 2001). Following are descriptions of some barriers to physical activity programming at the worksite and strategies for overcoming them.

■ *Some individuals do not want to exercise with their coworkers.* Worksite health promotion programs, including those that target physical activity, tend to attract only 20 to 30% of the workforce (Dishman et al., 1998). Following are several reasons people do not exercise at their worksites:

- For some, working out provides an escape from the stressors of the workplace; they do not want to increase their stress level by interacting with coworkers while exercising.
- Some people are embarrassed to sweat and work out in the presence of their coworkers.
- Some people prefer to work at work—not exercise or socialize.
- Workers often have many other competing interests that demand their time (e.g., family commitments, social pressures); thus they may perceive that working out at the worksite is too time intensive.

To overcome the barrier or stigma associated with exercising at work, program leaders should make programs and workout facilities highly attractive by offering unique and customized programs at convenient times, encouraging worksite competitions, and developing family-based worksite wellness programs.

■ *Some employees enjoy sedentary activities instead of active ones.* Some people would rather sit and read a book after work or watch TV than engage in physical activity. Therefore, program leaders should emphasize opportunities to multitask (e.g., read a book while riding a stationary cycle or watch TV while walking on a treadmill); this might educate previously sedentary people that they can multitask while exercising. Upper management can also consider installing treadmills or stationary bikes next to computers or offering physio balls in addition to regular office chairs.

Sample Successful Worksite-Based Physical Activity Programs

This section describes successful worksite physical activity programs. These programs are models for designing programs that are effective in the workplace.

Health Works for Women

Health Works for Women, developed by Tessaro and colleagues (2000), was an 18-month intervention that targeted 104 women in four small blue-collar worksites to improve a number of health behaviors including physical inactivity. The program was designed to follow the ecological model, in that multiple levels were targeted. Prior to the start of the intervention, focus groups were held to better understand participants' health concerns and address perceived barriers.

A key component and unique feature of Health Works for Women was that lay helpers were trained to deliver the program to their colleagues. Lay helpers were trained by nurses, nutritionists, and health educators, and training sessions were held onsite before or after work shifts for 45 to 90 minutes. The content of the training sessions included the role of support in making change, "female-specific issues" related to exercise, additional resources for health promotion in the local community, and skill building (including information about providing emotional support, listening, and problem solving). Upon completion of the training session, women leaders participated in a graduation ceremony, received T-shirts and tote bags, and were featured in an article published in the local press with photos.

The program was successful in that after 12 months, lay helpers were leading and organizing more activities. The most frequently led program was a walking group with coworkers at lunch or after work. Problems encountered were lack of time (e.g., overtime work schedules), conflicting work shifts, and after-work family obligations. This study was unique in that it featured information about training the trainers—a practice shown to be helpful in ensuring continued participation in the program.

Physical Activity Workplace Study (PAWS)

PAWS, developed by Plotnikoff and colleagues (2007), compared the efficacy of stage-matched materials (SM), standard materials (S), and a no-contact control condition (NCC) in terms of increasing physical activity in a Canadian workplace. Those in the SM group received a stage-matched book designed to target motivational readiness in each stage (contemplation, preparation, and action). Those in the S group received a two-page brochure with types and recommended amounts of physical activity and a 24-page handbook that contained information about the benefits of active living, problems with inactivity, how to choose physical activities that are right for them, and how to build activity into a routine. Those in the NCC group received no physical activity information, but came in for testing preintervention, at 6 months, and postintervention.

Although not statistically significant, a larger percentage of people in the SM group (19.3%) progressed from inactive to active from pre- to posttesting compared to those in the S group (11.7%) and the NCC group (15.4%). Additionally, there was a larger increase in MET-minutes (i.e., energy expenditure in METS multiplied by minutes of participation, a common term for quantifying participation in physical activity) of at least moderate-intensity physical activity in the SM group compared to the S and NCC groups (223, 78, and 67 MET-minutes, respectively). These differences, although not statistically significant, are potentially clinically meaningful given the major impact of moving from sedentary to some activity. Interestingly, the effects of the SM program were greater for women than they were for men.

Ten Grand Steps

Thomas and Williams (2006) developed Ten Grand Steps, a 6-week program to increase physical activity within specific worksites in Australia. All participants attended a baseline session that included information about the importance of physical activity for good health, the rationale for taking 10,000 steps daily, and how this program fits with the national physical activity guidelines. Participants received a pedometer at the initial session and were shown how to use the pedometer, along with a step count diary. An information booklet was provided that included hints to increase walking and goal-setting tips. Participants were sent regular e-mails to remind them of their goals and provide motivation and support.

Ten Grand Steps was successful in that more than 30% of the staff participated in the program. Approximately 70% of participants reported walking regularly throughout the program. Participants reported a 10% increase in their number of steps from pre- to posttest (8,501 steps per day to 9,374 steps per day). Impressively, those with the lowest baseline levels of physical activity were the ones who improved the most and were the most likely to maintain their walking program during the follow-up period. They were also very likely to include their family members in their walking programs. A follow-up questionnaire given to participants upon completing the program indicated that 97% of the participants thought the program was worthwhile, 65% reported making other changes in their physical activity habits, and 54% said the program increased their knowledge about physical activity. Respondents also mentioned that management support for the program aided the success of the program.

GETTING STARTED

Checklist for Developing a Successful Worksite-Based Program

❑ Secure the support of top-level management.

❑ Focus on modifiable risk factors.

❑ Tailor the program to the characteristics or needs of the workforce.

❑ Use behavior modification strategies to facilitate behavior change.

❑ Find ways to entice people to want to exercise with coworkers (e.g., provide a comfortable, clean, supportive, and convenient environment, offer unique or innovative programming—including family-based programming).

❑ Teach employees to multitask (e.g., read a book while riding a stationary bike or watch TV or type at a computer while walking on a treadmill).

Summary

Clearly, the setting of a physical activity program can affect participation. Factors that affect participation in physical activity are different at home compared to the worksite or a church setting. Attention to factors that contribute to success, as well as barriers to programs within these settings, will help program planners design better interventions. Additionally, knowledge about a variety of previously successful programs with a variety of populations can also help physical activity intervention specialists design more successful programs.

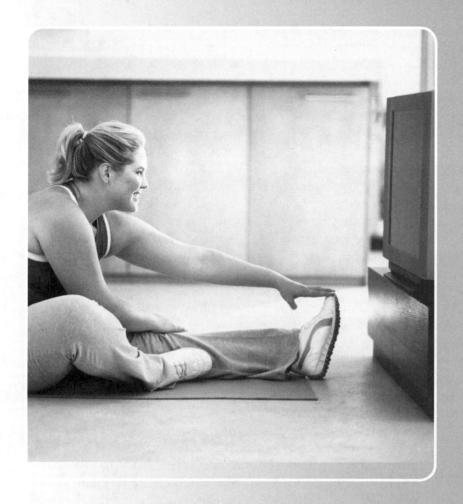

CHAPTER 10

Effectively Using Mediated Programming

Americans are becoming more and more technologically savvy. Most Americans have personal computers with Internet access and mobile phones. It is estimated that compared to 30 years ago, the average American spends 369 additional hours per year watching TV and 108 additional hours per year playing video games; this is a net gain of 2 hours per day in media consumption compared to life in 1977 (Mailbach, 2007). As the influence of technology continues to increase, those interested in promoting physical activity should consider developing physical activity programs that effectively use technology.

Using technology or intervention techniques that are not delivered face-to-face is known as mediated program delivery (Marshall, Owen, & Bauman, 2004). Because of the ability to reach large numbers of people with relatively low cost, mediated programs in our field have increased dramatically. Wantland, Portillo, Holzemer, Slaughter, and McGhee (2004) reported that during a 7-year period (1996-2003), there was a 12-fold increase in MEDLINE citations for "Web-based therapies." Some examples of mediated program delivery include using e-mail to contact program participants, using the Internet to track activity or seek social support or program feedback from group leaders, or offering podcasts or Web-streamed videos to provide access to important program information (Hurling et al., 2007; Wantland et al., 2004).

Mediated physical activity programs are attractive to program developers because they can be developed for a reasonable cost, and once they are developed, they typically cost less than mail- or phone-oriented programs (Sevick et al., 2007). Additionally, Americans love their computers and often work several hours a day on them. Using technology to deliver a physical activity intervention ensures a captive audience that is comfortable using a computer. Given the growth in technology, the ease with which computers can be used to influence physical activity behavior, and the level of success that has been recorded with previous mediated physical activity interventions (Dishman & Buckworth, 1996; Wantland et al., 2004), the purpose of this chapter is to do the following:

- Define and discuss various types of mediated interventions currently available
- Summarize the factors related to successful mediated physical activity interventions
- Discuss barriers to mediated physical activity interventions and strategies for overcoming them
- Highlight various aspects of some of the most successful programs to date

Types of Mediated Interventions

Marshall and colleagues (2004) classified mediated physical activity program delivery into four types: mass media, print, phone (including text messaging), and Web-based (including e-mail). Podcasts are also included as a type of mediated intervention. Like the other types of interventions, podcasts have the potential to make a significant impact, and they continue to increase in popularity.

■ *Mass media.* Mass media consists of large-scale television, radio, and newspaper advertisement or story coverage to promote physical activity. These campaigns typically use catchy slogans, slick advertising, and planned schedules of information delivery that target specific populations. Some examples of mass media campaigns to promote physical activity are Wheeling Walks, a promotional campaign for walking in West Virginia (Reger et al., 2002), and 10,000 Steps Rockhampton, a mass media campaign from Australia supported by community activities and environmental prompts (Brown, Eakin, Mummery, & Trost, 2003). The unique features of mass media are that it can serve as a supplementary strategy to other techniques, and it can occur at the national, state, or local level. Experts maintain that there is consistent evidence that mass media campaigns have a positive impact on the recall of campaign tag lines and message content, and that modest evidence suggests short-term impacts on behavior change in some population groups (Bauman, Bellew, Owen, & Vita, 2001; Marcus, Owen, Forsyth, Cavill, & Fridinger, 1998; Marshall et al., 2004). Figure 10.1 summarizes seven levels of impact (awareness, knowledge, saliency, attitudes, self-efficacy, intention, and behavior) that should be considered when using mass media to promote physical activity. Failure to consider all seven levels may result in an inability to reach the desired population.

■ *Print media.* Print media includes newspaper ads and stories, booklets, letters, and self-help brochures. Print media campaigns include the use of letters tailored to people's levels of motivation, readiness, or personality type (Marshall, Leslie, Bauman, Marcus, & Owen, 2003). These interventions are popular because they cost less than developing and maintaining Web sites or staffing phones for phone-based interventions (Sevick et al., 2007).

Marshall and colleagues (2004) suggested that the evidence to support the use of print media to facilitate physical activity behavior change is modest and that there is a need to develop supplemental strategies (e.g., establish frequency of contact recommendations and supplementary materials or additional modes of information delivery) to support print-based initiatives. Interestingly, some researchers purport that all delivery media are similar in terms of initiating increased physical activity; however, print media may be more effective than Web-based (Marcus, Lewis, et al., 2007; Marshall et al., 2003; Sevick et al., 2007) or telephone-based initiatives (Marcus, Lewis, et al., 2007) in terms of facilitating long-term changes in physical activity behavior. Following are some reasons print interventions may be more effective than other mediated delivery methods at facilitating long-term behavior change (Marks et al., 2006):

- Navigating through printed material is sometimes easier than navigating through material in other forms.

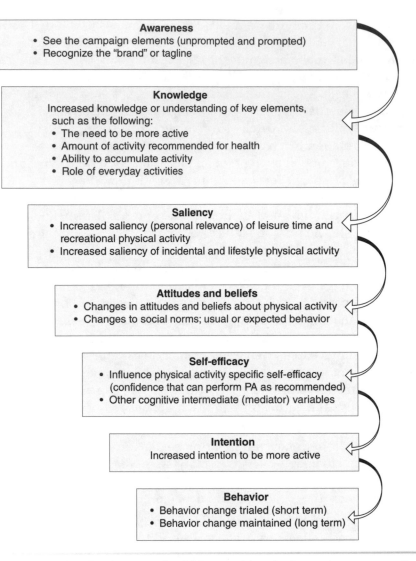

FIGURE 10.1 **Seven levels of impact should be considered when using mass media to promote physical activity.**

From N. Cavill and A. Bauman, 2004, "Changing the way people think about health-enhancing physical activity: Do mass media campaigns have a role?" *Journal of Sport Sciences* 22: 771-790. Reprinted by permission of the publisher (Taylor & Francis Ltd., http://www.tandf.co.uk/journals).

- Printed source documents are easier to annotate through highlighting or note taking than documents in other forms may be.

- There are no barriers to access with printed materials.

▪ *Phone-based initiatives.* These initiatives include phoning or text messaging those participating in a program to remind them to exercise, counsel them through difficult times (e.g., when they don't exercise because of time constraints or fatigue), and provide other information to help them succeed with their exercise program. Some examples of phone initiatives are fully automated phone counseling systems, text messaging to remind participants to exercise, and phone call follow-ups after completing an intervention. Experts agree that this area of research needs significantly more data prior to making conclusive statements about whether phone initiatives work (Marshall et al., 2004).

■ *Web-based initiatives.* These initiatives include using the Web to provide information, log exercise minutes, check on strategies for overcoming barriers, set exercise goals, and provide information about local community events. Marshall and colleagues (2003) suggested that Web-based initiatives have the following advantages over the print medium:

- Novelty
- Flexibility and convenience
- Interpersonal interaction
- Social support
- Ability to reach large numbers of people
- Data collected via the Internet are readily accessible and ready to use and interpret

Unfortunately, Web-based interventions can be costly initially (e.g., research and development fees), and Web maintenance issues cannot be ignored. Initial costs are comparable to developing other types of interventions, but in the long run, Web-based interventions may cost less than other types covered in this chapter (Marks et al., 2006; Sevick et al., 2007). Marshall and colleagues (2005) reported that survey respondents interested in receiving physical activity advice were quite interested in receiving information via the Internet and e-mail, so using the Web to increase physical activity is worth considering.

Because most previous studies targeted small, highly motivated groups who had frequent access to computers (Marshall et al., 2004), Web-based programming is an area of research that needs significantly more data prior to making conclusive statements about whether such initiatives work. Some very interesting new studies have tested whether interactive features (Hurling, Fairley, & Dias, 2006) on Web sites or theoretical fidelity to theories of behavior change (Rovniak, Hovell, Wojcik, Winett, & Martinez-Donate, 2005) increase the effectiveness of Web-based interventions.

■ *Podcasts.* A podcast is a relatively new method of disseminating information. Material that can be delivered via podcast includes news features, motivational speeches, interviews, presentations from conferences, debates, and workouts. Fitness professionals use them to supplement their face-to-face sessions, motivate clients, and market services (Hartman & Jackson, 2007). Podcasts are downloaded from the Internet onto a computer or portable music device such as an MP3 player or iPod. They contain dialogue as well as videos or photos. Podcasts cover specific topics, and listeners typically subscribe to them. Some organizations provide free podcasts, and others charge per download or per month. One major benefit of podcasting is that the down-loaded audio file can be listened to at one's convenience, including during a workout. Following are two Web sites that offer physical activity–related podcasts (Eads, 2007; Hartman & Jackson, 2007):

- www.itrain.com (fee-based)
- www.podcastdirectory.com/format/Fitness (mostly free fitness podcasts)

Factors Related to Successful Mediated Physical Activity Interventions

Factors related to successful mediated physical activity interventions fall into two categories: (a) general and relevant for all types of mediated interventions and (b) specific and relevant to only certain types of mediated interventions. Both are addressed in this section. Designers of interventions should consider both general and specific aspects when planning mediated programs.

General Factors Related to Success in All Mediated Interventions

The following six factors are related to success with any type of mediated intervention, regardless of medium:

- Increasing dose-response
- Designing memorable campaign slogans and information
- Using market segmentation and message personalization strategies
- Targeting multiple media outlets
- Ensuring theoretical fidelity
- Paying attention to quality control

■ *Dose-response issues.* Dose-response, in this context, means that more media exposure typically results in increased physical activity behavior, increased satisfaction with program components, or both. Mediated interventions, if used correctly, can reach large numbers of people in a cost-effective manner. Exposure to media is measured in weekly gross rating points (GRP). One GRP means that 1% of the target audience viewed the advertisement once. Obviously, higher GRPs are more likely to result in a successful campaign (i.e., reach large numbers of people).

■ *Memorable campaign slogans.* A second key to developing a successful mediated campaign is to develop and use memorable and reproducible images. Most people interested in physical activity will remember Nike's most memorable ad campaigns: "Just Do It," "If you let me play . . .," and the recent ads in conjunction with the women's World Cup soccer tournament ("The greatest team you've never heard of"). The average American is exposed to 3,000 ads per day (Peterson, Abraham, & Waterfield, 2005); therefore, media must be memorable to make an impact.

▪ *Market segmentation.* Market segmentation refers to designing marketing strategies for a specific segment of the population. Designing campaigns so they will reach various age or ethnic groups or men or women is an important strategy because what works for one segment of the population may be offensive or nonmeaningful to another (Peterson, Abraham, & Waterfield, 2005). To ensure memorable messages and accurate market segmentation, program promoters should pilot test campaign slogans and designs with the target audience. In addition to pilot testing, it is important to continually seek feedback, preferably from a local advisory committee, to refine and improve a media message as necessary. When possible, booster campaigns should be administered to sustain a promotional effort beyond the life of the initial campaign (Reger et al., 2002).

▪ *Personalization strategies.* Similar to market segmentation (or personalizing a message to reach a target audience), Marcus and colleagues (1998) suggested that one of the most important factors contributing to a successful mediated program is identifying and including relevant attributes of role models. For example, if a message is designed to reach young African Americans in a community, then characteristics and attributes of young African Americans and representative role models should be included in that message. To ascertain what these characteristics are and what information might be meaningful to that group, members of the relevant group should be surveyed and included in a pilot testing process. The bottom line is that if people can personalize a message, they are more likely to internalize and act on it. Additional factors that can help facilitate program success are (a) tailoring information to a specific stage of change (such as the contemplation stage in the transtheoretical model), (b) updating the stage of change regularly; and (c) using reinforcement letters, phone calls, or e-mails regularly (e.g., biweekly) (Marshall et al., 2003).

▪ *Targeting multiple areas of the media.* Numerous media outlets are available for health and fitness–related messages (e.g., billboards, buses, signs, television, radio, Internet, and newspaper) (Peterson et al., 2005). A good example of creative media blitzing is using point-of-decision prompts. Point-of-decision prompts are reminders in the form of signs, bulletin boards, billboards, or bus signs that encourage people to take advantage of physical activity opportunities when they arise (Marcus et al., 1998). Some examples of point-of-decision prompts that work include Use the Stairs and Park and Walk (Marcus et al., 1998).

▪ *Theoretical fidelity.* Theoretical fidelity refers to the precision with which theory-based recommendations are used. Rovniak and colleagues (2005) tested the effectiveness of high- and low-fidelity e-mail-based walking interventions in 65 sedentary adults, mostly women. One 12-week intervention, which demonstrated high fidelity to the social cognitive theory (SCT), used targeted skills, specific and hierarchical goals, and precise self-monitoring and feedback. The other intervention, which demonstrated low fidelity to the SCT, provided information (rather than modeling) to teach skills and did not provide ongoing self-monitoring and feedback. Several outcomes were monitored before and after the intervention, including a 1-mile (1.6 km) walk test of physical fitness, a log of walking behavior, and several measures of social cognitive theory (e.g., exercise self-efficacy, benefits and enjoyment of physical activity, goal setting, exercise planning, and social support). Compared to those in the low-fidelity group, those in the high-fidelity group completed more of their prescribed walking sessions and walked faster at posttest. Those in the high-fidelity group also reported greater program satisfaction and increased their goal setting and positive outcome expectations for walking more than twice as much as those in the low-fidelity group. Clearly, efforts to ensure theoretical fidelity are important for improving the success of mediated interventions.

▪ *Quality control.* Quality control, or attention to clarity, accuracy, and timeliness, is important. Information must be of high quality to earn respect, reach the critical mass, and facilitate changes in physical activity behavior (Marcus et al., 1998). Although obesity prevention and physical activity promotion are multimillion-dollar industries, it is not right to promise something that cannot be delivered. Failure to deliver programs based on factual information may result in an ineffective and disrespected program.

Factors Related to Success in Specific Mass Media Programs

The mass media has the potential to reach large numbers of people in a short period of time for a relatively low cost. To maximize this opportunity and ensure that mass media programs are successful, Cavill and Bauman (2004) recommend the following strategies:

- The mass media should target multiple media outlets in a systematic and sustained fashion.
- Campaigns should maximize contact or message exposure, because doing so typically results in greater behavior change.
- Other supportive community activities should be organized around mass media messages (e.g., self-help groups, counseling, screening and education, community events, and walking trails).
- The message coming from the mass media should be singular and simple—so it will be memorable.
- Mass media campaigns should target a specific audience or audiences based on demographics, attitudes, and preferred media usage; this will ensure that the message is heard by those for whom it is designed.

Print-Based Programs   Those designing physical activity programs are probably most familiar with print-based handouts. Print handouts have been around longer than other means of media, and they are probably still the most common method of promoting increased physical activity. Distributors of print media should use some of the suggestions provided earlier for all mediated interventions, while also considering specific recommendations for this medium. Following are some suggestions for designing a successful print-based program (Napolitano & Marcus, 2002):

- Follow up with participants quickly after distributing print material.
- Provide opportunities for participants to find interactions with others because social support is a desirable feature of many physical activity programs.
- Make sure the information is concise, accurate, and specifically directed to the targeted population.
- Pilot test materials with members of the targeted population.
- Write materials to a level appropriate for the targeted population.

Phone-Based Programs   Phone-based programs are delivered as phone calls or text messages. The following recommendations can help ensure that a phone-based program is successful:

- Consider the purpose of the contact (e.g., touching base, structured, or automated with prompts); studies have demonstrated that phone calls designed to touch base were just as effective as contacts that were highly structured (Lombard, Lombard, & Winett, 1995, as cited in Marcus et al., 1998).
- Consider the frequency with which phone calls or text messages are delivered. Schultz (1993) concluded that adherence and frequency of phone contacts are positively correlated, although there is probably a point at which a high frequency of phone contacts becomes a nuisance.
- Be as specific as possible with feedback (e.g., overcoming barriers, the benefits of exercise that are motivating to that participant, the type of activity the participant enjoyed) to facilitate maximal change (Hurling et al., 2007).

Although phone-based interventions have been around for a while, the use of text messaging to prompt physical activity is a relatively new means of communicating using mediated technology. Given the increase in text messaging in this country, this technology offers significant potential for reaching many people.

Web-Based Programs   Web-based programs demand a significant time investment prior to implementation. To ensure that Web-based programs are designed successfully, Ferney and Marshall (2006) recommended considering four factors that are important to Web site users in the field of physical activity promotion: Web design (structure), interactivity, environmental context, and content.

- *Web design.* To be maximally useful, Web sites should be easy to navigate and download time should be minimal (Ferney & Marshall, 2006). Users should be able to navigate a Web site easily, and links should be intuitive and downloadable in no more than 10 seconds. Making Web sites password protected facilitates tracking people's use around the site. Web site designers should conduct pilot and usability tests with proposed and developing Web sites and correct any problems found.

▪ *Interactivity.* A Web site that facilitates information exchange between a participant and an intervention specialist is interactive. Following are some examples of interactive activities on a PA Web site (Ferney & Marshall, 2006; Hurling et al., 2006):

- Logging on to a Web site to report activity or set goals
- Receiving specific feedback about one's performance compared to others or a previous best effort
- Accessing social support and expert advice
- Calculating target heart rate
- Accessing information about local community events
- Identifying barriers and receiving feedback about ways to overcome them

According to experts (Bull, Kreuter, & Scharff, 1999; Ferney & Marshall, 2006; Fogg, 2003; Hurling et al., 2006; Tate, Wing, & Winett, 2001; Wantland et al., 2004), interactive Web sites are more effective than noninteractive sites because they

- are more enjoyable to use,
- are less impersonal,
- facilitate better user retention and longer Web sessions,
- create higher expectations for exercise,
- facilitate higher levels of motivation and improved self-perception of fitness,
- are more likely to be saved and revisited in the future,
- are more likely to be discussed with others, and
- result in real behavior change with regular visitations.

▪ *Environmental context.* Providing information such as an updated community calendar of events; maps of physical activity opportunities in the community; and a physical activity database with information about times, costs, deadlines, and facilities (Ferney & Marshall, 2006) are examples of considering the environmental context. This information should be updated regularly to facilitate the desire to visit the Web site.

▪ *Content.* Information presented on the Web as audio, video, or text is known as content. It is important to update Web site content as often as possible. Those who use the Web frequently do not like to read volumes of text or wade through repetitive information, and they do not like to visit Web sites and see the same information over and over.

Podcasting Research is sparse on the factors related to success with podcasting—especially as it relates to increasing physical activity. However, until more research is conducted, the following basic strategies can help ensure that podcasts are successful (Eads, 2007; Hartman & Jackson, 2007):

- Be aware that those in the iPod generation are typically young and technologically savvy.
- When possible, provide the means for interaction with others.
- Pilot test podcasts with members of the target population.
- Make sure podcasts are simple and easy to download with a computer.

Barriers to Mediated Interventions and Strategies for Overcoming Them

An important barrier to mass media communication is the high cost of airtime (Cameron, Bauman, & Rose, 2006). Because television and radio stations can sell advertisements for large sums of money, their free public service announcements are limited. To overcome this barrier, program planners can use existing public service announcements, write grants to pay for airtime, or partner with other community or private groups to share costs. A barrier to print-based programming is the delay in receiving materials in the mail. To overcome this barrier, program planners can send information first class if possible and make information timely and attractive so the time delay will not influence the impact of the material.

Table 10.1. presents information on other barriers and strategies for overcoming them. Intervention specialists are encouraged to know as much as possible about barriers to participation so they can develop strategies for overcoming them.

TABLE 10.1 **Barriers to Successful Mediated Physical Activity Programs and Strategies for Overcoming Them**

Barrier and citation (if applicable)	Strategies for overcoming barrier
Mass media	
Cost of airtime; television, radio, and newspaper outlets can make more money on paid advertisements versus public service announcements (Cameron, Bauman, & Rose, 2006)	• Use public service announcement opportunities • Write grants to pay for airtime • Partner with other community or private groups to share costs • Use existing programs that have similar goals or outcomes
Communication is often complex and unpredictable (Faulkner & Finlay, 2006)	• Pilot test programs • Conduct process evaluations to assess program effectiveness • Form advisory committees to ensure that the message is effective

(continued) ▷

TABLE 10.1 *(continued)*

Barrier and citation (if applicable)	Strategies for overcoming barrier
Mass media	
Access to televisions, radios, and newspapers is limited in some parts of the world	• Provide increased access to media, if possible • Pilot test impact in populations where media outlets are limited
Cultural differences may not be effectively translated in media outlets	• Translate and back translate any media when possible • Use advisory committees to help determine whether program is culturally appropriate • Pilot test programs in small segments of the target population
Print-based media	
Cost of designing and printing materials	• As much as possible, use existing print resources • Partner with other community organizations to share costs
Delay in receiving materials as a result of mail services	• Send information first class if possible • Make information timely and attractive so time delay will not influence impact of material
Lack of interaction among participants and the program	• Provide suggestions for interaction opportunities such as worksheets, Web sites, interest groups, and activity opportunities
Phone-based media	
Cost of phone calls and text messaging	• Write grants to pay for cell phone minutes and text messages • Partner with other community or other private groups to share costs
Many parts of the world do not have access to phone technology	• Provide increased access to phone technology, if possible • Pilot test impact in populations where phone technology is limited
Web-based media	
Interest wanes quickly if Web site is not interactive (Marshall, Leslie, Bauman, Marcus, & Owen, 2003; Marshall, Owen, & Bauman, 2004)	• Design interactive Web-based programs that require participants to set goals, ask for expert advice, calculate resting and target exercise heart rates, access information about local community events, and identify barriers to their success • Include photos of program leaders interacting with participants on the Web site • Collect data on who uses the Web site and know when to make changes
High cost of developing and maintaining Web site	• Partner with other community groups to share costs • Write grants to support Web site development and maintenance

Barrier and citation (if applicable)	Strategies for overcoming barrier
Web-based media	
Some people (e.g., elderly, homeless, low income, or limited education) are intimidated by computers (Marcus et al., 1998; Wantland et al., 2004)	• Provide training sessions for those who are computer-phobic • Provide phone-based computer support for those who have questions about using computer technology
Podcasting	
Some people do not own or use computers or iPods regularly	• Write grants to provide technology for this population • Hold training sessions to familiarize participants with ways to download podcasts
Lack of interaction among participants and the program	• Provide suggestions for interaction opportunities such as worksheets, Web sites, interest groups, and activity opportunities

Sample Successful Mediated Interventions

To understand how to plan, implement, and evaluate mediated programming for physical activity, those responsible for designing programs should examine sample interventions. Some programs included multiple mediated strategies, and some compared media to see which was most successful in changing physical activity behavior. The programs outlined in the following sections demonstrate the use of a variety of mediated strategies.

10,000 Steps Rockhampton (Mass Media)

This 8-week campaign was developed in Queensland, Australia, to encourage people to take 10,000 steps per day (Brown et al., 2003). A secondary theme, "Every Step Counts," was added to the original notion of 10,000 steps to target those who might have difficulty meeting the 10,000-step recommendation. In contrast to a previous program that was very general (Active Australia, with the tagline, "Take it regularly—not seriously"), this program was designed to give people specific information to improve their health.

The designers of 10,000 Steps Rockhampton used five main strategies guided by the social-ecological framework: (a) organize a local media campaign, (b) promote activity through health care services (including from physicians), (c) improve social support for activity among disadvantaged groups, (d) design and implement policy and environmental approaches to increasing activity (e.g., encourage active transportation), and (e) establish small grant opportunities for community-level programming. Program activities included raising awareness of inactivity and profiling community role models, training people to conduct brief physical activity counseling, loaning pedometers to citizens and community groups on a trial basis, sending mail to dog owners, posting signage by trails, and sponsoring workplace competitions. Social support in disadvantaged groups was facilitated through community partners such as workplaces, the fitness industry, and the Heart Foundation (Australia's version of the American Heart Association).

The impact of this program is still being assessed, although increased physician counseling about physical activity has been reported in the intervention community (Eakin, Brown, Marshall, Mummery, & Larsen, 2004), as has increased pedometer usage and Web site visits (Eakin et al., 2007; Mummery, Schofield, Hinchliffe, Joyner, & Brown, 2006).

VERB Campaign (Mass Media)

The VERB campaign, funded for $194 million by the U.S. Centers for Disease Control and Prevention, was designed to use commercial marketing techniques to increase children's interest in healthful eating and physical activity (Huhman et al., 2007). The campaign was designed to spread the message that physical activity is cool, fun, and a chance to spend time with friends. TV advertisements were run on cable networks that kids watch, and activity promotion kits were given to community organizations and schools. An Activity Finder was included on the Web site so kids could locate physical activity opportunities by entering their zip codes. The effectiveness of the campaign was recently assessed in a large sample of parent–child dyads (n = 2,257). Outcome measures included psychosocial information (outcome expectations, self-efficacy, and social influences) and self-reported physical activity (free time and organized). There was a dose-response effect of exposure to the campaign: The more children saw the VERB messages, the more they participated in physical activity and demonstrated positive attitudes about activity.

Wheeling Walks (Mass Media)

The Wheeling Walks campaign used an 8-week program of mass media, public relations, and public health activities to improve awareness and attitudes and increase walking behavior in sedentary adults aged 50 to 65 years old (Reger et al., 2002). The mass media part of the program featured two newspaper ads, two 30-second television ads, and two 60-second radio ads. The primary goal of the program was to change the perception of behavioral control over exercise so that people who once thought they could not exercise because of time or other constraints could be convinced that they could not afford to be sedentary. Messages included: "Start walking 10 minutes a day, then 20 minutes" and "30 minutes of walking is the same amount of time it takes someone to watch 30 minutes of television." All ads ended with the tagline: "Isn't it time you started walking?" In addition to the media campaign, weekly press conferences and campaign events were featured on local news broadcasts, a Worksite Wellness Walking Challenge was held, a Web site was developed, and physicians were given pads of paper to write prescriptions for patients to walk 30 minutes or more, most days of the week.

The impact of the program was assessed using phone surveys in the intervention and comparison communities and observations of walkers at various sites throughout the two communities. As a result of the campaign, the number of walkers in the intervention community (as assessed by direct observation) increased by 23%, whereas the number of walkers in the comparison community decreased by 6%. Additionally, almost twice the number of people in the intervention community reported walking enough to meet the U.S. surgeon general's recommendation of 30 minutes, most days of the week (32%), compared to the community that did not receive the intervention (18%).

Fresh Start (Print)

This large study (n = 543) sought to compare the effects of a 10-month program of stage-specific mailed materials versus non-stage-specific (i.e., standardized health education products) materials in terms of increasing fruit and vegetable intake, increasing physical activity, and decreasing fat intake in a group of breast or prostate cancer survivors (Demark-Wahnefried et al., 2007). Both interventions received a personalized workbook and a series of seven newsletters at 6-week intervals. Regularly, between mailings, participants were asked to complete brief surveys for a small honorarium.

Participants in the stage-specific program received individually tailored materials based on stage of change (transtheoretical model) and reported barriers to changing health behaviors and progress toward goals. Information from the brief surveys was used to update modules. Participants in the non-stage-specific program received the "Facing Forward" booklet published by the National Cancer Institute and additional health education materials on eating a healthful diet and increasing exercise. Stage-specific and non-stage-specific programs resulted in increased exercise minutes per week, increased fruit and vegetable consumption, and decreased fat consumption. The unique features of this program were low attrition (4.4%), longitudinal data collection, multiple health behaviors targeted (e.g., physical activity and nutrition), and the use of mailed print interventions in a population that seeks to increase the likelihood of healthy survivorship after cancer.

Project STRIDE (Print and Phone)

Project STRIDE, developed by several of the leaders in physical activity interventions today, compared a phone-based intervention (PHB) to a print-based intervention (PRB) and contact control condition (CC) in terms of increasing initial physical activity and maintaining long-term participation in activity (Marcus, Napolitano, et al., 2007). PHB and PRB activities were based on assessing baseline stage of change from the transtheoretical model and using intervention activities that would facilitate movement through the stages of change. For example, people in the early stages of change (e.g., precontemplation, contemplation) may be more likely to respond to cognitive processes of change such as increasing awareness, whereas those in the later stages of change (e.g., preparation, action, and maintenance) may be more likely to respond to behavioral processes of change such as enlisting social support.

Messages, booklets, and tip sheets, based on stage of change, were generated by a computer expert system for participants in the PRB group. Participants in the PHB group received phone calls from a health educator, and those phone calls were directed by a computer expert system to ensure that feedback in both conditions was comparable. Contacts, numbering 14 over a period of 1 year, were more frequent at the beginning of the intervention and less frequent at the end.

At the end of 6 months, PHB and PRB groups experienced significant increases in minutes of moderate-intensity physical activity compared to the CC group. After 1 year, those in the PRB group reported significantly more minutes of moderate-intensity activity compared to their counterparts in the PHB and CC conditions. This indicates that both phone and print interventions facilitated short-term changes in physical activity, but the print medium may contribute more to long-term adherence. It is possible that the print medium is more effective because people can save and subsequently review materials. Interestingly, when usefulness of the program was assessed, participants rated phone calls as much more useful and supportive than print-based materials.

Active Living (Web and Print)

Active Living is an 8-week Web-based program that evolved from a print-based program (Marshall et al., 2003). This program assessed stage of change (according to the transtheoretical model) and featured personalized Web links to sites on goal setting, activity planning, and determining target heart rate. People who participated in this project were regularly reassessed to ensure that their Web information was tailored to their specific stage of change. The Web information was supplemented with personalized and stage-based reinforcement e-mails sent every 2 weeks. These e-mails contained hyperlinks to relevant areas of the Active Living Web site. The print information for this intervention was identical to the information found in the Web-based program except that people receiving the print materials received supplemental letters with stage-matched information every 2 weeks.

The impact of the intervention was assessed by comparing baseline and postintervention physical activity data: (a) MET-minutes per week and minutes in specific categories of activity (e.g., vigorous, moderate, and seated activities), collected with the International PA Questionnaire (IPAQ), (b) meeting or not meeting the public health recommendation (i.e., 30 minutes of at least moderate physical activity most days of the week), and (c) stage of change in the transtheoretical model. Results of the study indicate that Web intervention participants reported a decrease in the amount of time spent sitting, and print-based intervention participants increased their total minutes of physical activity. About 26% of the participants in both groups progressed forward at least one stage of change in the transtheoretical model, indicating that they should be likely to continue being physically active in the future. It is interesting to note that both print- and Web-based programs facilitated increases in physical activity, although people in the print group reported larger increases in activity and they were better able to recognize intervention materials after the program was completed.

America on the Move (Web)

One of the most creative Web-based programs for increasing physical activity is America on the Move. This program, available in Spanish or English, has intuitive appeal and has garnered significant interest in terms of mediated venues for increasing physical activity. Participants who log on to America-onthemove.org are asked to use pedometers to establish a baseline number of steps, increase their current level of physical activity by 2,000 steps per day, and eat 100 calories less per day. Competitions can be arranged between schools, work sites, businesses, churches, communities, and states. Some of the interesting and unique features of this Web site are (a) the ability to track the number of steps taken and apply them to progress on a famous American trail, (b) tips for decreasing caloric intake by 100 calories per day, (c) an opportunity to compare step counts to those of other people participating in the program across America, and (d) the opportunity to set goals and track progress.

Canada on the Move (Web)

Canada on the Move is a Web-based program sponsored by the Canadian Institutes of Health Research (CIHR) and Kellogg Canada (Dietz, 2006). In this program, 2 million pedometers were distributed in specially marked cereal boxes of Special K cereal, with instructions for using the pedometers and referral to the Canada on the Move Web site. The Web site was used to educate interested patrons as well as collect data to assess the impact of the pedometer distribution and promote walking behavior. Dissemination of this campaign information was limited because the number of people who had heard of the campaign increased by only 6%; however, recall of the specific message "Add 2,000 steps" increased threefold (Dietz, 2006). Awareness of pedometers increased substantially more than recall of the program name or Web-based slogans (Dietz, 2006), although there is some evidence of a dose-response relationship between the number of messages recalled and pedometer use (Craig, Cragg, Tudor-Locke, & Bauman, 2006). This program is unique in that it provides a positive example of passive dissemination of physical activity information, and it illustrates the potential of public–private community collaborations (Dietz, 2006).

Directions: This worksheet should be given to individuals involved in the planning process as well as a small sample of individuals from the desired population you plan to reach. The worksheet will be most effective if it is used during the pilot testing stages of a project. Information gleaned from this worksheet should be used to improve the project prior to full-scale implementation.

Questions	Yes	No	Suggested solutions
1. Were the materials **visually appealing**? If not, please add your suggestions in the box on the right.			
2. Were the materials **written or spoken at a level that is understandable** by a wide variety of people? If not, please add your suggestions in the box on the right.			
3. Did the materials **target a variety of media outlets** (e.g., TV, radio, newspaper, print, Web, podcasting)? If not, please write your suggestions in the box on the right.			
4. Were there any noticeable **barriers to accessing the information**? If yes, please write your suggestions for increasing access in the box on the right.			
5. Did the materials provide **opportunities for interacting with others**? If not, please write your suggestions for improving interactivity in the box on the right.			
6. Was there an **identifiable campaign slogan** and if so, was it memorable? If not, please write your suggestions for improving the impact of the slogan in the box.			
7. Was there evidence of **including theory in the program**? If not, please write your suggestions for improving the theoretical foundation of the program in the box on the right.			
8. Was the information **accurate and timely**? If not, please write your suggestions for improving the accuracy and timeliness in the box on the right.			
9. Was the information **personalized** (e.g., feedback, suggestions, tailored to participant needs)? If not, please write your suggestions for personalizing the program in the box on the right.			
10. Were **other community or private groups involved** in the planning or delivery of the program? If not, please write your recommendations for other community or private groups that might have an interest in this project in the box on the right.			
11. Was the **frequency of contact** with others planned? If not, please write your recommendations for frequency of contact in the box on the right.			

FIGURE 10.2 Worksheet for assessing the effectiveness of a mediated physical activity intervention.

From L. Ransdell, M. Dinger, J. Huberty, and K. Miller, 2009, *Developing Effective Physical Activity Programs* (Champaign, IL: Human Kinetics).

❏ Plan frequent contacts for maximal effectiveness (more contact = greater impact).

❏ Use multiple media outlets whenever possible to maximize impact.

❏ Become familiar with the types of mediated information delivery and try to match the desired population with specific mediated strategies when possible.

❏ Consider that these types of interventions require significant up-front financial and human costs compared to face-to-face interventions.

❏ Develop memorable campaign slogans to ensure that messages have an impact.

❏ Pilot test materials prior to releasing them to the desired population (figure 10.2 provides a checklist to use after pilot testing a program).

❏ As much as possible, maintain fidelity to theory-based recommendations.

❏ Deliver clear, accurate, and timely messages to earn respect.

❏ Make sure media messages match the reading, comprehension, and educational level of the desired audience.

❏ Maximize opportunities for interaction with mediated technology to sustain interest in the program and keep people motivated to pursue active lifestyles.

Summary

The use and impact of media in our society is continually increasing. Attempting to increase physical activity behavior using mediated methods is recommended because of the cost savings (especially when compared to labor-intensive, face-to-face programs) and the presence of the media in everyday life. Physical activity interventions using mediated delivery have had a significant impact on changing physical activity behavior (Dishman & Buckworth, 1996; Marshall, Owen, & Bauman, 2004). In all mediated programs, there are factors related to success and barriers with delivering mediated programs. The job of the physical activity promotion specialist is to enhance those factors related to success and minimize barriers to program adherence. To continue to use mediated techniques effectively, these specialists should evaluate these approaches more thoroughly—especially combinations of various types of mediated approaches.

REFERENCES

Preface

Ainsworth, B.E., Irwin, M.L., Addy, C.L., Whitt, M.C., & Stolarczyk, L.M. (1999). Moderate physical activity patterns of minority women: The cross-cultural activity participation survey. *Journal of Women's Health & Gender-Based Medicine, 8* (6), 805-813.

Allender, S. (2006). Understanding participation in sport and physical activity among children and adults: A review of qualitative studies. *Health Education Research, 21* (6), 826-835.

Caspersen, C.J., Powell, K.E., & Christenson, G.M. (1985). Physical activity, exercise, and physical fitness: Definitions and distinctions for health-related research. *Public Health Reports, 100* (2), 126-131.

U.S. Department of Health and Human Services (USDHHS). *Healthy People 2010: A midcourse review* (2005). Retrieved March 27, 2007, from www.healthypeople.gov/data/midcourse/pdf/fa22.pdf

Ransdell, L.B., Vener, J., & Sell, K. (2004). Gender and physical activity: International perspectives. *Journal of the Royal Society for Health, 124* (1), 12-14.

Introduction

Bock, B.C., Marcus, B.H., Pinto, B.M., & Forsyth, L.H. (2001). Maintenance of physical activity following an individualized motivationally tailored intervention. *Annals of Behavioral Medicine, 23* (2), 79-87.

Cox, K.L. (2003). Exercise behaviour change in 40- to 65-year-old women: The SWEAT Study (Sedentary Women Exercise Adherence Trial). *British Journal of Health Psychology, 8* (4), 477-495.

Dishman, R.K., & Buckworth, J. (1996). Increasing physical activity: A quantitative synthesis. *Medicine & Science in Sports & Exercise, 28* (6), 706-719.

Gittlesohn, J., Steckler, A., Johnson, C.C., Pratt, C., Grieser, M., Pickrel, J., Stone, E., Conway, T., Coombs, D., & Staten, L. (2006). Formative research in school and community-based health programs and studies: "State of the art" and the TAAG approach. *Health Education & Behavior, 33* (1), 25-39.

Glanz, K., Rimer, B.K., & Lewis, F.M. (Eds.). (2002). *Health behavior and health education* (3rd ed.). San Francisco: Jossey-Bass.

Pinto, B.M., Friedman, R., Marcus, B.H., Kelley, H., Tennstedt, S., & Gillman, M.W. (2002). Effects of a computer-based, telephone counseling system on physical activity. *American Journal of Preventive Medicine, 23* (2), 113-120.

Ransdell, L.B., Oakland, D., & Taylor, A. (2003). Increasing physical activity in girls and women: Lessons learned from the DAMET project. *Journal of Physical Education, Recreation, and Dance, 74* (1), 37-44, 55.

Chapter 1

Alcazar, O., Ho, R.C., & Goodyear, L.J. (2007). Physical activity, fitness, and diabetes mellitus. In C. Bouchard, S.N. Blair, & W.L. Haskell (Eds.), *Physical activity and health* (pp. 191-204). Champaign, IL: Human Kinetics.

American College of Sports Medicine. (2006). *ACSM's guidelines for exercise testing and prescription* (7th ed.). Baltimore, MD: Lippincott Williams & Wilkins.

Blair, S.N., & LaMonte, M.J. (2007). Physical activity, fitness, and mortality rates. In C. Bouchard, S.N. Blair, & W.L. Haskell, (2007). *Physical activity and health*. Champaign, IL: Human Kinetics.

Dunn, A.L., Trivedi, M.H., & O'Neal, H.A. (2001). Physical activity dose-response effects on outcomes of depression and anxiety. *Medicine & Science in Sports & Exercise, 33* (6 Suppl.), S587-597.

Haskell, W.L., Lee, I.M., Pate, R.R., Powell, K.E., Blair, S.N., Franklin, B.A., et al. (2007). Physical activity and public health: Updated recommendation for adults from the American College of Sports Medicine and the American Heart Association. *Medicine & Science in Sports & Exercise, 38* (8), 1423-1434.

Hootman, J. (2007). Physical activity, fitness, and joint and bone health. In C. Bouchard, S.N. Blair & W.L. Haskell (Eds.), *Physical activity and health* (pp. 219-230). Champaign, IL: Human Kinetics.

Institute of Medicine. (2005). *Dietary reference intakes for energy, carbohydrate, fiber, fat, fatty acids, cholesterol, protein, and amino acids (macronutrients).* Washington, DC: National Academy Press.

Institute of Medicine. (2007). *Adequacy of evidence for physical activity guidelines development: Workshop summary.* Washington, DC: National Academies Press.

Janssen, I. (2007). Physical activity, fitness, and cardiac, vascular, and pulmonary morbidities. In C. Bouchard, S.N. Blair & W.L. Haskell (Eds.), *Physical activity and health* (pp. 161-171). Champaign, IL: Human Kinetics.

Kelley, D.E., & Goodpaster, B.H. (2001). Effects of exercise on glucose homeostasis in type 2 diabetes mellitus. *Medicine & Science in Sports & Exercise, 33* (6 Suppl.), S495-S501.

Kesaniemi, Y.A., Danforth, E., Jensen, M.D., Kopelman, P.G., Lefebvre, P., & Reeder, B.A. (2001). Dose-response issues concerning physical activity and health: An evidence-based symposium. *Medicine & Science in Sports & Exercise, 33* (6), S345-S641.

Kohl, H.W. (2001). Physical activity and cardiovascular disease: Evidence for a dose response. *Medicine & Science in Sports & Exercise, 33* (6 Suppl.), S472-S483.

Kriska, A.M., & Caspersen, C.J. (1997). A collection of physical activity questionnaires for health-related research. *Medicine & Science in Sports & Exercise, 29* (6 Suppl.), S1-205.

Lee, I.M. (2007). Physical activity, fitness, and cancer. In C. Bouchard, S.N. Blair, & W.L. Haskell (Eds.), *Physical activity and health* (pp. 205-218). Champaign, IL: Human Kinetics.

Lee, I.M., & Skerrett, P.J. (2001). Physical activity and all-cause mortality: What is the dose-response relation? *Medicine & Science in Sports & Exercise, 33* (6 Suppl.), S459-S471.

Minino, A.M., Heron, M.P., Murphy, S.L., & Kochankek, K.D. (2007). *Deaths: Final data for 2004. National vital statistics reports.* Hyattsville, MD: National Center for Health Statistics.

Pate, R., Pratt, M., Blair, S., Haskell, W., Macera, C., Bouchard, C., et al. (1995). Physical activity and public health: A recommendation from the Centers for Disease Control and Prevention and the American College of Sports Medicine. *Journal of the American Medical Association, 273* (5), 402-407.

Raglin, J.S., Wilson, G.S., & Galper, D. (2007). Exercise and its effects on mental health. In C. Bouchard, S.N. Blair, & W.L. Haskell (Eds.), *Physical activity and health* (pp. 247-257). Champaign, IL: Human Kinetics.

Thune, I., & Furberg, A. (2001). Physical activity and cancer risk: Dose-response and cancer, all sites and site-specific. *Medicine & Science in Sports & Exercise, 33* (6 Suppl.), S530-S550.

U.S. Department of Health and Human Services. (1996). *Physical activity and health: A report of the surgeon general.* Atlanta, GA: U.S. Department of Health and Human Services, Centers for Disease Control and Prevention, National Center for Chronic Disease Prevention and Health Promotion.

U.S. Department of Health and Human Services. (2008). *2008 Physical Activity Guidelines for Americans.* Retrieved December 19, 2008, from www.health.gov/paguidelines.

U.S. Department of Health and Human Services & U.S. Department of Agriculture. (2005). *Dietary guidelines for Americans* (6th ed.). Washington, DC: U.S. Government Printing Office.

Vuori, I.M. (2001). Dose-response of physical activity and low back pain, osteoarthritis, and osteoporosis. *Medicine & Science in Sports & Exercise, 33* (6 Suppl.), S551-S586.

Chapter 2

Anspaugh, D.J., Dignan, M.B., & Anspaugh, S.L. (2006). *Developing health promotion programs* (2nd ed.). Long Grove, IL: Waveland Press.

Centers for Disease Control and Prevention. (2001). Increasing physical activity: A report on recommendations of the Task Force on Community Preventive Services. *Morbidity and Mortality Weekly Report, 50* (RR-18), 1-14.

Centers for Disease Control and Prevention. (2006). Increasing physical activity: Guide to Community Preventive Services Web site. Retrieved September 19, 2007, from www.thecommunityguide.org/pa/

Centers for Disease Control and Prevention. (2007a, July 16, 2007). Behavioral Risk Factor Surveillance System. Retrieved September 21, 2007, from www.cdc.gov/brfss/

Centers for Disease Control and Prevention. (2007b, August 22). National Health and Nutrition Examination Survey. Retrieved September 21, 2007, from www.cdc.gov/nchs/nhanes.htm

Green, L.W., & Kreuter, M.W. (2005). *Health program planning: An educational and ecological approach* (4th ed.). Boston: McGraw-Hill.

Green, L.W., & Lewis, F.M. (1986). *Measurement and evaluation in health education and health promotion*. Palo Alto, CA: Mayfield.

McKenzie, J.F., Neiger, B.L., & Smeltzer, J.L. (2005). *Planning, implementing & evaluating health promotion programs* (4th ed.). San Francisco, CA: Pearson Benjamin Cummings.

Task Force on Community Preventive Services. (2005). *The guide to community preventive services: What works to promote health?* New York: Oxford University Press.

U.S. Department of Health and Human Services. (1999). *Promoting physical activity: A guide for community action*. Champaign, IL: Human Kinetics.

U.S. Department of Health and Human Services. (2000). *Healthy People 2010* (2nd ed.). Washington, DC: U.S. Government Printing Office.

U.S. Department of Health and Human Services. (2002). *Physical activity evaluation handbook*. Atlanta, GA: U.S. Department of Health and Human Services, Centers for Disease Control and Prevention.

Chapter 3

Ainsworth, B.E. (2000a). Challenges in measuring physical activity in women. *Exercise and Sport Sciences Reviews, 28* (2), 93-96.

Ainsworth, B.E. (2000b). Practical assessment of physical activity. In K.A. Tritschler (Ed.), *Barrow & McGee's practical measurement and assessment* (pp. 475-492). Baltimore, MD: Lippincott Williams & Wilkins.

Ainsworth, B.E., Bassett, D.R., Strath, S.J., Swartz, A.M., O'Brien, W.L., Thompson, R.W., et al. (2000). Comparison of three methods for measuring the time spent in physical activity. *Medicine & Science in Sports & Exercise, 32* (9), S457-S464.

Ainsworth, B.E., Haskell, W.L., Whitt, M.C., Irwin, M.L., Swartz, A.M., Strath, S.J., et al. (2000). Compendium of physical activities: An update of activity codes and MET intensities. *Medicine & Science in Sports & Exercise, 32* (9 Suppl.), S498-S516.

Ainsworth, B.E., Jacobs, Jr., D.R., & Leon, A.S. (1993). Validity and reliability of self-reported physical activity status: the Lipid Research Clinics questionnaire. *Medicine & Science in Sports & Exercise, 25* (1), 92-98.

Baecke, J.A.H., Burema, J., & Frijters, J.E.R. (1982). A short questionnaire for the measurement of habitual physical activity in epidemiological studies. *American Journal of Clinical Nutrition, 36*, 936-942.

Bassett, D.R. (2000). Validity and reliability issues in objective monitoring of physical activity. *Research Quarterly for Exercise and Sport, 71* (2), 30-36.

Bassett, D.R., Schneider, P.L., & Huntington, G.E. (2004). Physical activity in an old order Amish community. *Medicine & Science in Sports & Exercise, 36* (1), 79-85.

Behrens, T.K., & Dinger, M.K. (2007). Motion sensor reactivity in physically active young adults. *Research Quarterly for Exercise and Sport, 78* (1), 1-8.

Buchowski, M.S., Acra, S., Majchrzak, K.M., Sun, M., & Chen, K.Y. (2004). Patterns of physical activity in free-living adults in the Southern United States. *European Journal of Clinical Nutrition, 58* (5), 828-837.

Caspersen, C.J., Powell, K.E., & Christenson, G.M. (1985). Physical activity, exercise, and physical fitness: Definitions and distinctions for health-related research. *Public Health Reports, 100* (2), 127-131.

Craig, C.L., Marshall, A.L., Sjostrom, M., Bauman, A.E., Booth, M.L., Ainsworth, B.E., et al. (2003). International Physical Activity Questionnaire: 12-country reliability and validity. *Medicine & Science in Sports & Exercise, 35* (8), 1381-1395.

Crouter, S.E., Clowers, K.G., & Bassett, D.R. (2006). A novel method for using accelerometer data to predict energy expenditure. *Journal of Applied Physiology, 100*, 1324-1331.

Crouter, S.E., Schneider, P.L., Karabulut, M., & Bassett, D.R. (2003). Validity of 10 electronic pedometers for measuring steps, distance, and energy cost. *Medicine & Science in Sports & Exercise, 35* (8), 1455-1460.

Dinger, M.K., & Behrens, T.K. (2006). Accelerometer-determined physical activity of free-living college students. *Medicine & Science in Sports & Exercise, 38* (4), 774-779.

Dinger, M.K., Heesch, K.C., & McClary, K.R. (2005). Feasibility of a minimal contact intervention to promote walking among insufficiently active women. *American Journal of Health Promotion, 20* (1), 2-6.

DuVall, C., Dinger, M.K., Taylor, E.L., & Bemben, D. (2004). Minimal-contact physical activity interventions in women: A pilot study. *American Journal of Health Behavior, 28* (3), 280-286.

Godin, G., & Shephard, R.J. (1985). A simple method to assess exercise behavior in the community. *Canadian Journal of Applied Sport Sciences, 10* (3), 141-146.

Jacobs, D.R., Hahn, L.P., Haskell, W.L., Pirie, P., & Sidney, S. (1989). Reliability and validity of a short physical activity history: CARDIA and the Minnesota Health Program. *Journal of Cardiopulmonary Rehabilitation, 9*, 448-459.

Kriska, A.M., & Caspersen, C.J. (1997). A collection of physical activity questionnaires for health-related research. *Medicine & Science in Sports & Exercise, 29* (6 Suppl.), S1-205.

Kriska, A.M., Knowler, W.C., LaPorte, R.E., Drash, A.L., Wing, R.R., Blair, S.N., et al. (1990). Development of questionnaire to examine relationship of physical activity and diabetes in Pima Indians. *Diabetes Care, 13* (4), 401-411.

Matevey, C., Rogers, L.Q., Dawson, E., & Tudor-Locke, C. (2006). Lack of reactivity during pedometer self-monitoring in adults. *Measurement in Physical Education and Exercise Science, 10* (1), 1-11.

Matthews, C.E., Ainsworth, B., Thompson, R.W., & Bassett, D.R. (2002). Sources of variance in daily physical activity levels as measured by an accelerometer. *Medicine & Science in Sports & Exercise, 34* (8), 1376-1381.

Montoye, H.J. (1971). Estimation of habitual physical activity by questionnaire and interview. *American Journal of Clinical Nutrition, 24*, 1113-1118.

Pate, R., Pratt, M., Blair, S., Haskell, W., Macera, C., Bouchard, C., et al. (1995). Physical activity and public health: A recommendation from the Centers for Disease Control and Prevention and the American College of Sports Medicine. *Journal of the American Medical Association, 273* (5), 402-407.

Sallis, J.F., Haskell, W.L., Wood, P.D., Fortmann, S.P., Rogers, T., Blair, S.N., et al. (1985). Physical activity assessment in the five-city project. *American Journal of Epidemiology, 121* (1), 91-106.

Sallis, J.F., & Saelens, B.E. (2000). Assessment of physical activity by self-report: Status, limitations, and future directions. *Research Quarterly for Exercise and Sport, 71* (2), 1-14.

Schneider, P.L., Crouter, S.E., & Bassett, D.R. (2004). Pedometer measures of free-living physical activity: Comparison of 13 models. *Medicine & Science in Sports & Exercise, 36* (2), 331-335.

Sequeira, M.M., Rickenbach, M., Wietlisbach, V., Tullen, B., & Schutz, Y. (1995). Physical activity assessment using a pedometer and its comparison with a questionnaire in a large population survey. *American Journal of Epidemiology, 142*, 989-999.

Shapiro, S., Weinblatt, E., Frank, C.W., & Sager, R.V. (1969). Incidence of coronary heart disease in a population insured for medical care (HIP). *American Journal of Public Health and the Nation's Health, 59* (6 Suppl.), 1-101.

Taylor, H.L., Jacobs, D.R., Shucker, B., Knudsen, J., Leon, A.S., & DeBacker, G. (1978). A questionnaire for the assessment of leisure-time physical activities. *Journal of Chronic Diseases, 31*, 741-755.

Troiano, R.P. (2005). A timely meeting: Objective measurement of physical activity. *Medicine & Science in Sports & Exercise, 37* (11 Suppl.), S487-S489.

Trost, S.G., McIver, K.L., & Pate, R.R. (2005). Conducting accelerometer-based activity assessments in field-based research. *Medicine & Science in Sports & Exercise, 37* (11 Suppl.), S531-543.

Tudor-Locke, C., & Bassett, D.R. (2004). How many steps/day are enough? *Sports Medicine, 34* (1), 1-8.

Tudor-Locke, C., Bassett, D.R., Swartz, A.M., Strath, S.J., Parr, B.B., & Reis, J.P. (2004). A preliminary study of one year of pedometer self-monitoring. *Annals of Behavioral Medicine, 28*, 158-162.

Tudor-Locke, C., Bell, R.C., Myers, A.M., Harris, S.B., Lauzon, N., & Rodger, N.W. (2002). Pedometer-determined ambulatory activity in individuals with type 2 diabetes. *Diabetes Research and Clinical Practice, 55*, 191-199.

Tudor-Locke, C., & Myers, A.M. (2001). Methodological considerations for researchers and practitioners using pedometers to measure physical (ambulatory) activity. *Research Quarterly for Exercise and Sport, 72* (1), 1-12.

Ward, D.S., Evenson, K.R., Vaughn, A., Rodgers, A.B., & Troiano, R.P. (2005). Accelerometer use in physical activity: Best practices and research recommendations. *Medicine & Science in Sports & Exercise, 37* (11 Suppl.), S582-588.

Washburn, R.A., Smith, K.W., Jette, A.M., & Janney, C.A. (1993). The Physical Activity Scale for the Elderly (PASE): Development and evaluation. *Journal of Clinical Epidemiology, 46* (2), 153-162.

Wilde, B.E., Sidman, C.L., & Corbin, C.B. (2001). A 10,000-step count as a physical activity target for sedentary women. *Research Quarterly for Exercise and Sport, 72* (4), 411-414.

Chapter 4

Albright, C.L., Pruitt, L., Castro, C., Gonzalez, A., Woo, S., & King, A.C. (2005). Modifying physical activity in a multiethnic sample of low-income women: One-year results from the impACT (Increasing Motivation for Physical ACTivity) project. *Annals of Behavioral Medicine, 30* (3), 191-200.

Anton, S.D., Perri, M.G., Riley, J., Kanasky, W.F., Rodrigue, J.R., Sears, S.F., & Martin, A.D. (2005). Differential predictors of adherence in exercise programs with moderate versus higher levels of intensity and frequency. *Journal of Sport and Exercise Psychology, 27* (2), 171-187.

Benn, T. (2006). Incompatible? Compulsory mixed-sex physical education initial teacher training and the inclusion of Muslim women: A case study on seeking solutions. *European Physical Education Review, 12* (2), 181-200.

Brassington, G.S., Atienza, A.A., Perczek, R.E., Dilorenzo, T.M., & King, A.C. (2002). Intervention-related cognitive versus social mediators of exercise adherence in the elderly. *American Journal of Preventive Medicine, 23* (2S), 80-86.

Courneya, K.S., & McAuley, E. (1995). Cognitive mediators of the social influence-exercise adherence relationship: A test of the theory of planned behavior. *Journal of Behavioral Medicine, 18* (5), 499-515.

Cox, K.L., Burke, V., Gorely, T.J., Beilin, L.J., & Puddey, I.B. (2003). Controlled comparison of retention and adherence in home- vs. center-initiated exercise interventions in women ages 40-65 years: The SWEAT Study (Sedentary Women Exercise Adherence Trial). *Preventive Medicine, 36* (1), 17-29.

Cramp, A.G. & Brawley, L.R. (2006). Moms in Motion: A community based cognitive behavioral physical activity intervention. *International Journal of Behavioral Nutrition and Physical Activity, 3* (23), 1-9.

Dacey, M., Baltzell, A., & Zaichkowsky, L. (2003). Factors in women's maintenance of vigorous or moderate physical activity. *Women in Sport and Physical Activity Journal, 12* (1), 87-111.

Derry, J.A. (2002). Single-sex and coeducational physical education: Perspectives of adolescent girls and female physical education teachers. *Melpomene Journal, 21* (3), 21-28.

Duncan, G.E. (2006). Exercise, fitness, and cardiovascular disease risk in type 2 diabetes and the metabolic syndrome. *Current Diabetes Reports, 6* (1), 29-35.

Ekkekakis, P., & Lind, E. (2006). Exercise does not feel the same when you are overweight: The impact of self-selected and imposed intensity on affect and exertion. *International Journal of Obesity, 30* (4), 652-660.

Eyler, A.E., Wilcox, S., Matson-Koffman, D., Evenson, K.R., Sanderson, B., Thompson, J., Wilbur, J., & Rohm-Young, D. (2002). Correlates of physical activity among women from diverse racial/ethnic groups. *Journal of Women's Health & Gender-Based Medicine, 11* (3), 239-253.

Farris, R.P., Haney, D.M., & Dunet, D.O. (2004). Expanding the evidence for health promotion: Developing best practices for WISEWOMAN. *Journal of Women's Health, 13* (5), 634-643.

Finkenberg, M.E., Dinucci, J., McCune, S.L., Chenette, T., & McCoy, P. (1998). Commitment to physical activity and anxiety about physique among college women. *Perceptual and Motor Skills, 87* (3, pt. 2), 1393-1394.

Huberty, J.L., Ransdell, L.B., Sidman, C., Flohr, J.A., Shultz, B., Grosshans, O., & Durrant, L. (2008). Explaining long-term exercise adherence in women who complete a structured exercise program. *Research Quarterly for Exercise and Sport, 79* (3), 374-384.

Jakicic, J.M., Winters, C., Lang, W., & Wing, R.R. (1999). Effects of intermittent exercise and use of home exercise equipment on adherence, weight loss, and fitness in overweight women. *Journal of the American Medical Association, 282* (16), 1554-1560.

Jeon, C.Y., Lokken, R.P., Hu, F.B., & van Dam, R.M. (2007). Physical activity of moderate intensity and risk of type 2 diabetes: A systematic review. *Diabetes Care, 30* (3), 744-752.

Kugler, J., Seelbach, H., & Kruskemper, G.M. (1994). Effects of rehabilitation exercise programs on anxiety and depression in coronary patients: A meta-analysis. *The British Journal of Clinical Psychology, 33* (pt. 3), 401-410.

Lemmon, C.R., Ludwig, D.A., Howe, C.A., Ferguson-Smith, A., & Barbeau, P. (2007). Correlates of adherence to a physical activity program in young African-American girls. *Obesity, 15* (3), 695-703.

Marcus, B.H., Napolitano, M.A., King, A.C., Lewis, B.A., Whiteley, J.A., Albrecht, A.E., Parisi, A.F., Bock, B.C., Pinto, B.M., Sciamanna, C.A., Jakicic, J.M., & Papandonatos, G.D. (2007). Telephone versus print delivery of an individualized motivationally tailored physical activity intervention: Project STRIDE. *Health Psychology, 26* (4), 401-409.

Martyn-St. James, M., & Carroll, S. (2006). High-intensity resistance training and postmenopausal bone loss: A meta-analysis. *Osteoporosis International, 17* (8), 1225-1240.

McAuley, E., Jerome, G.J., Marquez, D.X., Elavsky, S., & Blissmer, B. (2003). Exercise self-efficacy in older adults: Social, affective, and behavioral influences. *Annals of Behavioral Medicine, 25* (1), 1-7.

McKenzie, T.L., Prochaska, J.J., Sallis, J.F., & LaMaster, K.J. (2004). Coeducational and single-sex physical education in middle schools: Impact on physical activity. *Research Quarterly for Exercise & Sport, 75* (4), 446-449.

Napolitano, M.A., Papandonatos, G.D., Lewis, B.A., Whiteley, J.A., Williams, D.M., King, A.C., Bock, B.C., Pinto, B., & Marcus, B.H. (2008). Mediators of physical activity behavior change: A multivariate approach. *Health Psychology, 27* (4), 409-418.

Nies, M., Vollman, M., & Cook, T. (1999). American women's experiences with physical activity in their daily lives. *Public Health & Nursing, 16*, 23-31.

Oka, R.K., King, A.C., & Young, D.R.(1995). Sources of social support as predictors of exercise adherence in women and men ages 50 to 65 years. *Women's Health: Research on Gender, Behavior, and Policy, 2*, 161-175.

Oman, R.F., & King, A.C. (1998). Predicting the adoption and maintenance of exercise participation using self-efficacy and previous exercise participation rates. *American Journal of Health Promotion, 12* (3), 154-161.

Osuji, T., Lovegreen, S., Elliott, M., & Brownson, R.C. (2006). Barriers to physical activity among women in the rural Midwest. *Women & Health, 44* (1), 41-55.

Pate, R.R., Ward, D.S., Saunders, R.P., Felton, G., Dishman, R.K., & Dowda, M. (2005). Promotion of physical activity among high school girls: A randomized controlled trial. *American Journal of Public Health, 95* (9), 1582-1587.

Ransdell, L.B., Oakland, D., & Taylor, A. (2003a). Increasing physical activity in girls and women: Lessons learned from the DAMET project. *Journal of Physical Education, Recreation, and Dance, 74* (1), 37-44, 55.

Ransdell, L.B., Robertson, L., Ornes, L., & Moyer-Mileur, L. (2004). Generations exercising together to improve fitness (GET FIT): A pilot study designed to increase physical activity and improve health-related fitness in three generations of women. *Women & Health, 40* (3), 79-96.

Ransdell, L.B., Taylor, A., Oakland, D., Schmidt, J., Moyer-Mileur, L., & Shultz, B. (2003b). Daughters and mothers exercising together: Effects of home- and community-based programs. *Medicine & Science in Sports & Exercise, 35* (2), 286-296.

Ransdell, L.B., Vener, J., & Sell, K. (2004). Gender and physical activity: International perspectives. *Journal of the Royal Society for Health, 124* (1), 12-14.

Sallis, J., Hovell, M., & Hofstetter, C. (1992). Predictors of adoption and maintenance of vigorous physical activity in men and women. *Preventive Medicine, 21*, 237-251.

Scharff, D., Homan, S., Krueter, M., & Brennan, L. (1999). Factors associated with physical activity in women across the lifespan: Implications for program development. *Women & Health, 29*, 115-134.

Stoddard, A.M., Palombo, R., Troped, P.J., Sorensen, G., & Will, J.C. (2004). Cardiovascular disease risk reduction: The Massachusetts WISEWOMAN project. *Journal of Women's Health, 13* (5), 539-546.

U.S. Department of Health and Human Services (USDHHS). *Healthy People 2010: A midcourse review* (2005). Retrieved March 27, 2007, from www.healthypeople.gov/data/midcourse/pdf/fa22.pdf

White, J.L., Ransdell, L.B., Vener, J., & Flohr, J.A. (2005). Factors related to physical activity adherence in women: Review and suggestions for future research. *Women & Health, 41* (4), 123-148.

Wilbur, J., Miller, A.M., Chandler, P., & McDewitt, J. (2003). Determinants of physical activity and adherence to a 24-week home based walking program in African American and Caucasian women. *Research in Nursing & Health, 26*, 213-224.

Will, J.C., Farris, R.P., Sanders, C.G., Stockmyer, C.K., & Finkelstein, E.A. (2004). Health promotion interventions for disadvantaged women: Overview of the WISEWOMAN projects. *Journal of Women's Health, 13* (3), 484-502.

Yancy, A.K., McCarthy, W.J., Harrison, G.G., Wong, W.K., Siegel, J.M., & Leslie, J. (2006). Challenges in improving fitness: Results of a community-based, randomized, controlled lifestyle change intervention. *Journal of Women's Health, 15* (4), 412-429.

Chapter 5

Ainsworth, B.E., Haskell, W.L., Leon, A.S., Jacobs, D.R., Montoye, H.J., Sallis, J.F., & Paffenbarger, R.S. (1993). Compendium of physical activities: Classification of energy costs of human physical activities. *Medicine & Science in Sports & Exercise, 25* (1), 71-80.

American College of Sports Medicine (ACSM). (2006). *ACSM's guidelines for exercise testing and prescription* (7th ed.). Baltimore, MD: Lippincott Williams & Wilkins.

Anderson, J.W., Konz, E.C., Frederich, R.C., & Wood, C.L. (2001). Long-term weight loss maintenance: A meta-analysis of US studies. *American Journal of Clinical Nutrition, 74* (5), 579-584.

Andreyeva, T., Michaud, P.C., & van Soest, A. (2007). Obesity and health in Europeans aged 50 years and older. *Public Health, 121*, 497-509.

Ash, S., Reeves, M., Bauer, J., Dover, T., Vivanti, A., Leong, C., O'Moore-Sullivan, T., & Capra, S., (2006). A randomized control trial comparing lifestyle groups, individual counseling, and written information in the management of weight and health outcomes over 12 months. *International Journal of Obesity, 30*, 1557-1564.

Baum, C.G., & Forehand, R. (1984). Social factors associated with adolescent obesity. *Journal of Pediatric Psychology, 9* (3), 293-302.

Bellizzi, M.C., & Dietz, W.H. (1998). Workshop on childhood obesity: Summary of the discussion. *American Journal of Clinical Nutrition, 70* (1 pt. 2), 173S-175S.

Berger, B.G., Motl, R.W., Martin, D.T., Wilkinson, J.G., & Owen, D.R. (1999). Mood and cycling performance in response to three weeks of high intensity, short duration overtraining and a two week taper. *Sport Psychologist, 13*, 466-479.

Byrne, N.M., Meerkin, J.D., Laukkanen, R., Ross, R., Fogelholm, M., & Hills, A.P. (2006). Weight loss strategies for obese adults: Personalized weight management program vs. standard care. *Obesity, 14*, 1777-1788.

Caballero, B. (2004). Obesity prevention in children: Opportunities and challenges. *International Journal of Obesity, 28*, S90-S95.

Calle, E.E., & Kaaks, R. (2004). Overweight, obesity and cancer: Epidemiological evidence and proposed mechanisms. *National Reviews of Cancer, 4* (8), 579-591.

Carey, W.B., Hegvik, R.L., & McDevitt, S.C. (1988). Temperamental factors associated with rapid weight gain and obesity in middle childhood. *Journal of Developmental and Behavioral Pediatrics, 9* (4), 194-198.

Centers for Disease Control and Prevention. (2007). Obesity and overweight. Retrieved May 27, 2007, from www.cdc.gov/nccdphp/dnpa/obesity/economic_consequences.htm

Chehab, L.G., Pfeffer, B., Vargas, I., Chen, S., & Irigoyen, M. (2007). "Energy Up": A novel approach to the weight management of inner-city teens. *Journal of Adolescent Health, 40*, 474-476.

Colditz, G.A., Willett, W.C., Rotnitzky, A., & Manson, J.E. (1995). Weight gain as a risk factor for clinical diabetes mellitus in women. *Annals of Internal Medicine, 122* (7), 481–486.

Curioni, C.C., & Lourenco, P.M. (2005). Long-term weight loss after diet and exercise: A systematic review. *International Journal of Obesity, 29* (10), 1168-1174.

Deitel, M. (2003). Overweight and obesity worldwide now estimated to involve 1.7 billion people. *Obesity Surgery, 13*, 329-330.

Ekkekakis, P., & Lind, E. (2006). Exercise does not feel the same when you are overweight: The impact of self-selected and imposed intensity on affect and exertion. *International Journal of Obesity, 30*, 652-660.

Fiore, H., Travis, S., Whalen, A., Auinger, P., & Ryan, S. (2006). Potentially protective factors associated with healthful body mass index in adolescents with obese and nonobese parents: A secondary data analysis of the Third National Health and Nutrition Examination Survey, 1988-1994. *Journal of the American Dietetic Association, 106* (1), 55-64.

Fowler-Brown, A., & Kahwati, L.C. (2004). Prevention and treatment of overweight in children and adolescents. *American Family Physician, 69*, 2591-2598.

Garrow, J.S., & Summerbell, C.D. (1995). Meta-analysis: Effect of exercise, with or without dieting, on the body composition of overweight subjects. *European Journal of Clinical Nutrition, 49* (1), 1-10.

Gillison, F.B., Standage, M., & Skevington, S.M. (2006). Relationship among adolescents' weight perceptions, exercise goals, exercise motivation, quality of life, and leisure time exercise behaviour: A self-determination theory approach. *Health Education Research 21* (6), 836-847.

Hedley, A.A., Ogden, C.L., Johnson, C.L., Carroll, M.D., Curtin, L.R., & Flegal, K.M. (2004). Prevalence of overweight and obesity among U.S. children, adolescents, and adults, 1999-2002. *Journal of the American Medical Association, 291* (23), 2847-2850.

Huang, Z., Willett, W.C., Manson, J.E., Rosner, B., Stampfer, M.J., Speizer, F.E., & Colditz, G. (1998). Body weight, weight change, and risk for hypertension in women. *Annals of Internal Medicine, 128* (2), 81-88.

Jakicic, J.M., & Otto, A.D. (2006). Treatment and prevention of obesity: What is the role of exercise? *Nutrition Reviews, 64* (2, pt. 2), S57-S61.

Janssen, I., Katzmarzyk, P.T., Boyce, W.F., Vereecken, C., Mulvihill, C., Roberts, C., et al. (2005). Health behavior in school-aged children Obesity Working Group. Comparison of overweight and obesity prevalence in school-aged youth from 34 countries and their relationships with physical activity and dietary patterns. *Obesity Reviews, 6*, 123-132.

Kaur, H., Hyder, M., & Poston, W.S.C. (2003). Childhood overweight: An expanding problem. *Treatments in Endocrinology, 2* (6), 375-388.

Klem, M.L., Wing, R.R., McGuire, M.T., Seagle, H.M., & Hill, J.O. (1997). A descriptive study of individuals successful at long-term maintenance of substantial weight loss. *American Journal of Clinical Nutrition, 66*, 239-246.

Kuczmarski, R.J., Ogden, C.L., Grummer-Strawn, L.M., Flegal, K.M., Guo, S.S., Wei, R., Mei, Z., Curtin, L.R., Roche, A.F., & Johnson, C.L. (2000). CDC growth charts: United States. *Advance Data, Jun 8* (314), 1-27. (Also retrieved May 27, 2007, from www.cdc.gov/growthcharts)

Manson, J.E., Bassuk, S.S., Hu, F.B., Stampfer, M.J., Colditz, G.A., & Willett, W.C. (2007). Estimating the number of deaths due to obesity: Can the divergent findings be reconciled? *Journal of Women's Health, 16* (2), 168-176.

Mathus-Vliegen, E.M. (2007). Long-term health and psychosocial outcomes from surgically induced weight loss: Results obtained in patients not attending protocolled follow-up visits. *International Journal of Obesity, 31* (2), 299-307.

Miller, W.C., Koceja, D.M., & Hamilton, E.J. (1997). A meta-analysis of the past 25 years of weight loss research using diet, exercise or diet plus exercise intervention. *International Journal of Obesity and Related Metabolic Disorders, 21* (10), 941-947.

National Center for Health Statistics (NCHS) Health E-Stats. (2008). *Prevalence of overweight and obesity among adults: United States, 1999-2002.* Retrieved June 19, 2008, from www.cdc.gov/nchs/products/pubs/pubd/hestats/obese/obse99.htm

National Heart, Lung, and Blood Institute (NHLBI). (1998). Clinical guidelines on the identification, evaluation, and treatment of overweight and obesity in adults—The Evidence Report. Washington, DC: NIH Publication Number 98-4083.

National Weight Control Registry. (2007). Retrieved May 26, 2007, from www.nwcr.ws/

Neumark-Sztainer, D. (2005). Preventing the broad spectrum of weight-related problems: Working with parents to help teens achieve a healthy weight and a positive body image. *Journal of Nutrition Education and Behavior, 37,* S133-S139.

Neumark-Sztainer, D., Kaufmann, N.A., & Berry, E.M. (1995). Physical activity within a community-based weight control program: Program evaluation and predictors of success. *Public Health Reviews, 23,* 237-251.

Nothwehr, F., Snetselaar, L., & Wu, H. (2006). Weight management strategies reported by rural men and women in Iowa. *Journal of Nutrition Education & Behavior, 38,* 249-253.

Olshansky, S.J., Passaro, D.J., Hershow, R.C., Layden, J., Carnes, B.A., Brody, J., Hayflick, L., Butler, R.N., Allison, D.B., & Ludwig, D.S. (2005). A potential decline in life expectancy in the United States in the 21st century. *New England Journal of Medicine, 352* (11), 1138-1145.

Othersen-Gorman, M. (1999, February). Making the connection. *Runner's World,* 42-51.

Palmeira, A.L., Teixeira, P.J., Branco, T.L., Martins, S.S., Minderico, C.S., Themudo, J.L., Serpa, S.O., & Sardinha, L.B. (2007). Predicting short-term weight loss using four leading health behavior change theories. *International Journal of Behavioral Nutrition and Physical Activity, 4,* 14-41.

Parfitt, G., Rose, E.A., & Burgess, W.M. (2006). The psychological and physiological responses of sedentary individuals to prescribed and preferred intensity exercise. *British Journal of Health Psychology, 11,* 39-53.

Puhl, R.M., & Brownell, K.D. (2006). Confronting and coping with weight stigma: An investigation in overweight and obese adults. *Obesity, 14* (10), 1802-1815.

Rexrode, K.M., Hennekens, C.H., Willett, W.C., Colditz, G.A., Stampfer, M.J., Rich-Edwards, J.W., Speizer, F.E., & Manson, J.E. (1997). A prospective study of body mass index, weight change, and risk of stroke in women. *Journal of the American Medical Association, 277* (19), 1539-1545.

Segar, M., Spruijt-Metz, D., & Nolen-Hoeksema, S. (2006). Go figure? Body-shape motives as associated with decreased physical activity participation among midlife women. *Sex Roles, 54* (3/4), 175-187.

Shaw, K., O'Rourke, P., Del Mar, C., & Kenardy, J. (2005). Psychological interventions for overweight or obesity. Cochrane database of systematic reviews (CD003818). Retrieved May 23, 2007, from www.cochrane.org/reviews/en/ab003818.html

Snethen, J.A., Broome, M.E., & Cashin, S.E. (2006). Effective weight loss for overweight children: A meta-analysis of intervention studies. *Journal of Pediatric Nursing, 21* (1), 45-56.

Thomas, H. (2006). Obesity prevention programs for children and youth: Why are their results so modest? *Health Education Research, 21* (6), 783-795.

van Wier, M.F., Ariëns, G.A., Dekkers, J.C., Hendriksen, I.J., Pronk, N.P., Smid, T., & van Mechelen, W. (2006). ALIFE@Work: a randomised controlled trial of a distance counselling lifestyle programme for weight control among an overweight working population. *BMC Public Health, 6,* 140.

Weight Control Information Network. (2007). Retrieved May 27, 2007, from http://win.niddk.nih. gov/index.htm

World Health Organization. (2008). Obesity and overweight. Retrieved June 19, 2008, from www. who.int/dietphysicalactivity/publications/facts/obesity/en/

Willett, W.C., Manson, J.E., Stampfer, M.J., Colditz, G.A., Rosner, B., Speizer, F.E., & Hennekens, C.H. (1995). Weight, weight change, and coronary heart disease risk in women: Risk within the "normal" weight range. *Journal of the American Medical Association, 273* (6), 461-465.

You, T., Murphy, K.M., Lyles, M.F., Demons, J.L., Lenchik, L., & Nichlas, B.J. (2006). Addition of aerobic exercise to dietary weight loss preferentially reduces abdominal adipocyte size. *International Journal of Obesity, 30* (8), 1211-1216.

Chapter 6

American College of Sports Medicine (ACSM). (2006). *ACSM's guidelines for exercise testing and prescription* (7th ed.). Baltimore, MD: Lippincott Williams & Wilkins.

Baker, K.R., Nelson, M.E., Felson, D.T., Layne, J.E., Sarno, R., & Roubenoff, R. (2001). The efficacy of home based progressive strength training in older adults with knee osteoarthritis: A randomized controlled trial. *Journal of Rheumatology, 28* (7), 1655-1665.

Benjamin, K., Edwards, N.C., & Baharti, V.K. (2005). Attitudinal, perceptual, and normative beliefs influencing the exercise decisions of community-dwelling physically frail seniors. *Journal of Aging and Physical Activity, 13,* 276-293.

Booth, M.L., Owen, N., Bauman, A., Clavisi, O., & Leslie, E. (2002). Social-cognitive and perceived environmental influences associated with physical activity in older Australians. *Preventive Medicine, 31,* 15-22.

Brawley, L.R., Rejeski, W.J., & King, A.C. (2003). Promoting physical activity for older adults. *American Journal of Preventive Medicine, 25* (3Sii), 172-183.

Brawley, L.R., Rejeski, W.J., & Lutes, L. (2000). A group-mediated cognitive behavioral intervention for increasing adherence to physical activity in older adults. *Journal of Applied Biobehavioral Research, 5* (1), 47-65.

Brassington, G.S., Atienza, A.A., Perczek, R.E., DiLorenzo, T.M., & King A.C. (2002). Intervention-related cognitive versus social mediators of exercise adherence in the elderly. *American Journal of Preventive Medicine, 23* (2S), 80-86.

Campbell, A.J., Robertson, M.C., Gardner, M.M., Norton, R.N., & Buchner, D.M. (1999). Falls prevention over 2 years: A randomized controlled trial in women 80 years and older. *Age and Ageing, 28,* 513-518.

Canadian Society for Exercise Physiology Expert Advisory Committee. (2002). *Physical activity readiness questionnaire.* Ottawa, ON: Canadian Society for Exercise Physiology.

Cohen-Mansfield, J., Marx, M.S., & Guralnick, J.M. (2003). Motivators and barriers to exercise in an older community-dwelling population. *Journal of Aging and Physical Activity, 11,* 242-253.

Elley, C.R., Kerse, N., Aarol, B., & Robinson, E. (2003) Effectiveness of counseling patients on physical activity in general practice: Cluster randomized controlled trial. *BMJ (Clinical research ed.), 326* (12), 793-796.

Ettinger, W.H., Burns, R., Messier, S.P., Applegate, W., Rejeski, W.J., Morgan, T., et al. (1997). A randomized trial comparing aerobic exercise and resistance exercise with a health education program in older adults with knee osteoarthritis: The fitness arthritis and seniors trial (FAST). *Journal of the American Medical Association, 277* (1), 25-42.

Gill, T.M., Baker, D.I., Gottschalk, M., Reduzzi, P/N., Allore, H., & Byers, A. (2002). A program to prevent functional decline in physically frail elderly persons who live at home. *New England Journal of Medicine, 347* (14) 1068-1074.

Hays, K.A., & Clark, D.O. (1999). Correlates of physical activity in a sample of older adults with type 2 diabetes. *Diabetes Care, 22,* 706-712.

Jones, J.R., Jakobi, J.M., Taylor, A.W., Petrella, R.J., & Vandervoort, A.A. (2006). Community exercise program for older adults recovering from hip fracture: A pilot study. *Journal of Aging and Physical Activity, 14,* 439-455.

King, A.C., Haskell, W.J., Taylor, C.B., Kraemer, H.C., & Debusk, R.F. (1991). Group- vs. home-based exercise training in healthy older men and women: A community-based trial. *Journal of the American Medical Association, 266* (11), 535-543.

King, A.C., Haskell, W. J., Young, D.R., Oka, R.K., & Stefanic, M.L. (1995). Long-term effects of varying intensities and formats of physical activity on participation rates, fitness, and lipoproteins in men and women aged 50 to 65 years. *Circulation, 91* (10), 2596-2604.

King, A.C., Pruitt, L.A., Phillips, W., Oka, R., Rodenburg, A., & Haskell, W.L. (2000). Comparative effects of two physical activity programs on measured and perceived physical functioning and other health related quality of life outcomes in older adults. *Journal of Gerontology: MEDICAL SCIENCES, 55A* (2) M74-M83.

Lee, Y.S., & Laferty, S.C. (2006). Predictors of physical activity in older adults with borderline hypertension. *Nursing Research, 55* (2), 110-120.

Lees, F.D., Clark, P.G., Nigg, C.R., & Newman, P. (2005). Barriers to exercise behavior among older adults: A focus-group study. *Journal of Aging and Physical Activity, 13*, 23-33.

Litt, M.D., Kleppinger, A., & Judge, J.O. (2002). Initiation and maintenance of exercise behavior in older women: Predictors from the social learning model. *Journal of Behavioral Medicine, 25 (1)*, 83-97.

McAuley, E., Jerome, G.J., Elavvsky, S., Marquez, D.X., & Ramsey, S.N. (2003). Predicting long-term maintenance of physical activity in older adults. *Preventive Medicine, 37*, 110-118.

McMurdo, M.E., & Rennie, L. (1993). A controlled trial of exercise by residents of old people's homes. *Age and Ageing, 22*, 11-15.

Messier, S.P., Royer, T.D., Craven, T.E., O'Toole, M.L., Burns, R., & Ettinger, W.H. (2000). Long-term exercise and its effect on balance in older, osteoarthritic older adults: Results from the Fitness, Arthritis, and Seniors Trial (FAST). *Journal of the American Geriatrics Society, 48*, 131-138.

National Center for Health Statistics. (2004). *Reports from the 2004 National Health Interview Survey, Series10 No. 228*. Retrieved September 27, 2007, from www.cdc.gov/nchs/about/major/nhis/reports_2004.htm

Navarro, J.E., Sanz, J.L.G., del Castillo, J.M., Izquierdo, A C., & Rodriguez, M.M. (2007). Motivational factors and physical advice for physical activity in older urban adults. *Journal of Aging and Physical Activity, 15* (3), 241-256.

Rasinaho, M., Herninalo, M., Leinonen, R., Linutenen, T., & Rantinen, T. (2006). Motives for and barriers to physical activity among older adults with mobility limitations. *Journal of Aging and Physical Activity, 15*, 90-102.

Rejeski, W.J., & Brawley, L.R. (2006). Functional health: Innovations in research on physical activity with older adults. *Medicine & Science in Sports & Exercise, 38* (1), 93-99.

Rejeski, W.J., Brawley, L.R., Ambrosius, W.T., Brubaker, P.H., Focht, B.C., Foy, C.D., & Fox, L.D. (2003). Older adults with chronic disease: Benefits of group-mediated counseling in the promotion of physically active lifestyles. *Health Psychology, 22* (4), 414-423.

Resnick, B. (2002). Testing the effect of the WALC intervention on exercise adherence in older adults. *Journal of Gerontological Nursing, 28* (6), 40-49.

Resnick, B., Orwig, D., Magaziner, J., & Wynne C. (2002). The effect of social support on exercise behavior in older adults. *Clinical Nursing Research, 11* (1), 52-70.

Schutzer, K.A., & Graves, B.S. (2004). Barriers and motivations to exercise in older adults. *Prevention Medicine, 39*, 1056-1061.

Stevens, J.A., Corso, P.S., Finkelstein, E.A., & Miller, T.R. (2006). The costs of fatal and non-fatal falls among older adults. *Injury Prevention, 12*, 290-295.

Stewart, A.L., Mills, K.M., Sepis, P.G., King, A.C., McLellen, B.Y., Roita, K., et al. (1997). Evaluation of CHAMPS, a physical activity promotion program for older adults. *Annals of Behavioral Medicine, 19* (4), 353-361.

Stewart, A.L., Verboncoeur, C.J., McLellan, B.Y., Gillis, D.E., Rush, S., Mills, K.M., et al. (2001). Physical activity outcomes of CHAMPS II: A physical activity promotion program for older adults. *Journal of Gerontology: MEDICAL SCIENCES, 56A* (8), M465-M470.

Stuart, C.L., Marret, J., Kelly, G.A., & Nelson, R. (2002). Predictors of physical activity in older adults in an independent living retirement community. *The American Journal of Geriatric Cardiology, 11* (3), 160-164.

Taylor A.H., Cable, N.T., Faukner, G., Hillsdon, M., Narici, M., & van dir Bij, A.K. (2004). Physical activity and older adults: A review of health benefits and the effectiveness of interventions. *Journal of Sports Sciences, 22*, 703-725.

U. S. Census Bureau. (2004). U.S. interim projections by age, sex, race, and Hispanic origin. Retrieved September 27, 2007, from www.census.gov/ipc/usinterimproj/

U.S. Department of Health and Human Services. (1996). *Physical activity and health: A report of the surgeon general (executive summary).* Pittsburgh, PA: Superintendent of Documents.

U.S. Department of Health and Human Services. (2005). Leisure time physical activity by age, sex, and race/ethnicity. Retrieved September 27, 2007, from http:// 209.217.72.34/aging/Table Viewer/ tableView.aspx?reportID = 383

van der Bij, A.K., Laurant, M.G., & Wensing, M. (2002). Effectiveness of physical activity interventions for older adults. *American Journal of Preventive Medicine, 22* (2), 120-133.

Chapter 7

Ainsworth, B.E., Irwin, M.L., Addy, C.L., Whitt, M.C., & Stolarczyk, L.M. (1999). Moderate physical activity patterns of minority women: The cross-cultural activity participation study. *Journal of Women's Health & Gender Based Medicine, 8* (6), 805-813.

Albright, C.L., Pruitt, L., Castro, C., Gonzalez, A., Woo, S., & King, A.C. (2005). Modifying physical activity in a multiethnic sample of low-income women: one-year results from the impACT (Increasing Motivation for Physical ACTivity) Project. *Annals of Behavioral Medicine, 30* (3), 191-200.

Anderson, E.S., Wojcik, J.R., Winett, R.A., & Williams, D.M. (2006). Social-cognitive determinants of physical activity: The influence of social support, self-efficacy, outcome expectations, and self-regulation among participants in a church-based health promotion study. *Health Psychology, 25* (4), 510-520.

Bachar, J.J., Lefler, L.J., Reed, L., McCoy, T., Bailey, R., & Bell, R. (2006). Cherokee choices: A diabetes prevention program for American Indians. *Preventing Chronic Disease.* Retrieved June 2007 from www.cdc.gov/pcd/issues/2006/jul/05_0221.htm

Banks-Wallace, J., & Conn, V. (2002). Interventions to promote physical activity among African American women. *Public Health Nursing Research, 19* (5), 321-335.

Belza, B., Walwick, J., Shiu-Thornton, S., Schwartz, S. Taylor, M., & LoGerfo, J. (2004). Older adult perspectives on physical activity and exercise: Voices from multiple cultures. *Preventing Chronic Disease.* Retrieved June 2008 from http://www.cdc.gov/pcd/issues/2004/oct/04_0028.htm

Bopp, M., Lattimore, D., Wilcox, S., Laken, M., McClorin, L., Swinton, R., Gethers, O., & Bryant, D. (2006). Understanding physical activity participation in members of an African American church: A qualitative study. *Health Education and Research, 22* (6), 815-826.

Centers for Disease Control. (2004). Physical activity among Asians and native Hawaiians or other Pacific Islanders—50 states and the District of Columbia, 2001-2003. *Morbidity and Mortality Weekly Reports, 53* (33), 756-760.

Centers for Disease Control. (2005). Health data for all ages. U.S. Department of Health and Human Services. Retrieved June 4, 2007, from http://209.217.72.34/HDAA/TableViewer/chartVIEW. aspx

Chen, A.H., Sallis, J.F., Castro, C.M., Lee, R.E., Hickmann, S.A., Williams, C., & Martin, J.E. (1998). A home-based behavioral intervention to promote walking in sedentary ethnic minority women: Project Walk. *Women's Health: Research on Gender, Behavior, and Policy, 4* (1), 19-39.

Coble, J.D., & Rhodes, R.E. (2006). Physical activity and Native Americans: A review. *American Journal of Preventive Medicine, 31* (1), 36-46.

Coleman, K.J., & Gonzalez, E.C. (2001). Promoting stair use in a U.S.-Mexico border community. *American Journal of Public Health, 91* (12), 2007-2009.

Collins, R., Lee, R.E., Albright, C.L., & King, A.C. (2004). Ready to be physically active? The effects of a course preparing low-income multi-ethnic women to be more physically active. *Health Education & Behavior, 31* (1), 47-64.

Crespo, C.J. (2000). Encouraging physical activity in minorities. *The Physician and Sports Medicine, 28* (10). Accessed June 6, 2007, from www.physsportsmed.com/issues/2000/10_00/crespo.htm

Doshi, S.R., & Jiles, R. (2006). Health behaviors among American Indian/Alaska Native women, 1998-2000 BRFSS. *Journal of Women's Health, 15* (8), 919-927.

Escobar-Chavez, S.L., Tortolero, S.R., Masse, L.C., Watson, K.B., & Fulton, J.E. (2002). Recruiting and retaining minority women: Findings from the Women on the Move study. *Ethnicity and Disease, 12* (2), 242-251.

Evenson, K.R., Sarmiento, O.L., Macon, M.L., Tawney, K.W., & Ammerman, A.S. (2002). Environmental, policy, and cultural factors related to physical activity among Latina immigrants. *Women and Health, 36* (2), 43-57.

Eyler, A.A., Baker, E., Cromer, L., King, A.C., Brownson, R.C., & Donatelle, R.J. (1998). Physical activity and minority women: A qualitative study. *Health Education & Behavior, 25* (5), 640-652.

Eyler, A.A., Matson-Koffman, D., Vest, J.R., Evenson, K.R., Sanderson, B., Thompson, J.L., Wilbur, J., Wilcox, S., & Young, D.R. (2002). Environmental, policy, and cultural factors related to physical activity in a diverse sample of women: The women's cardiovascular health network project—introduction and methodology. *Women and Health, 36* (2), 1-15.

Eyler, A.A., Matson-Koffman, D., Vest, J.R., Evenson, K.R., Sanderson, B., Thompson, J.L., Wilbur, J., Wilcox, S., & Young, D.R. (2002). Environmental, policy, and cultural factors related to physical activity in a diverse sample of women: The women's cardiovascular health network project—summary and discussion. *Women and Health, 36* (2), 123-134.

Grassi, K., Gonzalez, M.G., Tello, P., & He, G. (1999). La Vida Caminando: A community-based physical activity program designed by and for rural Latino families. *Journal of Health Education, 30* (2), S13-S17.

Heesch, K.C., & Masse, L.C. (2004). Lack of time for physical activity: Perception or reality for African American and Hispanic women. *Women and Health, 39* (3), 45-62.

Heesch, K.C., Brown, D.R., & Blanton, C.J. (2000). Perceived barriers to exercise and stage of exercise adoption in older women of different racial and ethnic groups. *Women and Health, 30* (4), 61-76.

Juarbe, T., Turok, X.T., & Perez-Stable, E.J. (2002). Perceived benefits and barriers to physical activity among older Latina women. *Western Journal of Nursing Research, 24* (8), 868-886.

Kreuter, M.W., Lukwago, S.N., Bucholtz, D.C., Clark, E.M., & Sanders-Thomson, V. (2002). Achieving cultural appropriateness in health promotion programs: Targeted and tailored approaches. *Health Education & Behavior, 30* (2), 133-146.

Kurian, A.K., & Cardarelli, K.M (2007). Racial and ethnic differences in cardiovascular disease risk factors: A systematic review. *Ethnicity & Disease, 17* (1), 143-152.

Lee, S. (2005). Physical activity among minority populations: What health promotion practitioners should know—A commentary. *Health Promotion Practice, 6,* 447-452.

Mampilly, C.M., Yore, M.M., Maddock, J.E., Nigg, C.R., Buchner, D., & Heath, G.W. (2005). Prevalence of physical activity levels by ethnicity among adults in Hawaii, BRFSS 2001. *Hawaii Medical Journal, 64* (10), 272-273.

Marcus, B.H., Williams, D.M., Dubbert, P.M., Sallis, J.F., King, A.C., Yancey, A.K., Franklin, B.A., Buchner, D., Daniels, S.R., & Clayton, R.P. (2006). Physical activity intervention studies: What we know and what we need to know: A scientific statement from the American Heart Association Council on Nutrition, Physical Activity, and Metabolism (subcommittee on Physical Activity); Council on Cardiovascular Disease in the Lung; and the Interdisciplinary Working Group of Quality of Care and Outcomes Research. *Circulation, 114,* 2739-2752.

Masse, L.C., Ainsworth, B.E., Tortolero, S., Levin, S., Fulton, J.E., Henderson, K.A., & Mayo, K. (1998). Measuring physical activity in midlife, older, and minority women: Issues from an expert panel. *Journal of Women's Health, 7* (1), 57-67.

Maxwell, A.E., Bastani, R., Vida, P., & Warda, U.S. (2002). Physical activity among older Filipino-American women. *Women Health, 36* (1), 67-79.

Ransdell, L.B., & Rehling, S.L. (1996). Church-based health promotion: A review of the current literature. *American Journal of Health Behavior, 20* (4), 195-207.

Sriskantharajah, J., & Kai, J. (2007). Promoting physical activity among South Asian women with coronary heart disease and diabetes: What might help? *Family Practitioner, 24* (1), 71-76.

Staten, L.K., Gregory-Mercado, K.Y., Ranger-Moore, J., Will, J.C., Giuliano, A.R., Ford, E.S., & Marshall, J. (2004). Provider counseling, health education, and community health workers: The Arizona WISEWOMAN project. *Journal of Women's Health, 13* (5), 547-556.

Stoddard, A.M., Palombo, R., Troped, P.J., Sorensen, G., & Will, J.C. (2004). Cardiovascular disease risk reduction: The Massachusetts WISEWOMAN project. *Journal of Women's Health, 13* (5), 539-546.

U.S. Department of Health and Human Services. (2003). Physical activity among adults: United States. Retrieved June 11, 2007, from www.hhs.gov/news/press/2003pres/20030514.html

Wang, C.Y., Abbott, L., Goodbody, A.K., Hui, W.Y., & Rausch, C. (1999). Development of a community-based diabetes management program for Pacific Islanders. *The Diabetes Educator, 25* (5), 738-746.

Whitehorse, L.E., Manzano, R., Baezconde-Garbanati, L.A., & Hahn, G. (1999). Culturally tailoring a physical activity program for Hispanic women: Recruitment successes of La Vida Beuna's salsa aerobics. *Journal of Health Education, 30* (2), S18-S24.

Wilbur, J., Chandler, P., Dancy, B., Choi, Ji Won, & Plonczynski, D. (2002). Environmental, policy, and cultural factors related to physical activity in urban, African American women. *Women & Health, 36* (2), 17-28.

Wilbur, J., Miller, A.M., Chandler, P., & McDevitt, J. (2003). Determinants of physical activity and adherence to a 24-week home-based walking program in African American and Caucasian women. *Research in Nursing and Health, 26,* 213-224.

Yancey, AK., McCarthy, W.J., & Leslie, J. (1998). Recruiting African-American women to community-based health promotion research. *American Journal of Health Promotion, 12,* 335-338.

Yancey, A.K., Miles, O., & Jordan, A.D. (1999). Organizational characteristics facilitating initiation and institutionalization of physical activity programs in a multi-ethnic urban community. *Journal of Health Education, 30* (2), S44-S51.

Yancey, A.K., Jordan, A., Bradford, J., Voas, J., Eller, T.J., Buzzard, M., Welch, M., & McCarthy, W.J. (2003). Engaging high-risk populations in community-level fitness promotion: ROCK! Richmond. *Health Promotion Practice, 4* (2), 180-188.

Yancey, A.K., Kumanyika, S.K., Ponce, N.A., McCarthy, W.J., Fielding, J.E., Leslie, J.P., & Akbar, J. (2004). Population-based interventions engaging communities of color in healthy eating and active living: A review. *Preventing Chronic Disease.* Retrieved June 2007 from www.cdc.gov/pck/issues/2004/jan/03_0012.htm

Young, D.R., He, X., Harris, J., & Mabry, I. (2002). Environmental, policy, and cultural factors related to physical activity in well-educated urban African American women. *Women and Health, 36* (2), 29-41.

Chapter 8

Addy, C.L., Wilson, D.K., Kirtland, K.A., Ainsworth, B.E., Sharpe, P., & Kimsey, D. (2004). Associations of perceived social and physical environmental supports with physical activity and walking behavior. *American Journal of Public Health, 94* (3), 440-443.

Ainsworth, B.E., Wilcox, S., Thompson, W.W., Richter, D.L., & Henderson, K.A. (2003). Personal, social, and physical environmental correlates of physical activity in African-American women in South Carolina. *American Journal of Preventive Medicine, 25* (3), 23-29.

American College of Sports Medicine (ACSM). (1998). The recommended quantity and quality of exercise for developing and maintaining cardiorespiratory and muscular fitness, and flexibility in healthy adults. *Medicine & Science in Sports & Exercise, 30,* 975-991.

Berrigan, D., & Troiano, R.P. (2002). The association between urban form and physical activity in U.S. adults. *American Journal of Preventive Medicine 23* (2S), 74-79.

Boutelle, K.N., Jeffery R.W., Murray, D.M., & Schmitz, M.K.H. (2001). Using signs, artwork, and music to promote stair use in a public building. *American Journal of Public Health, 91* (12), 2004-2006.

Brownson, R.C., Baker, E.A., Boyd, R.L., Caito, N.M., Duggan, K., Housemann, R.A., Krueter, M.W., Mitchell, T., Motton, F., Pulley, C., Schmid, T.L., & Walton, D. (2004). A community-based approach to promoting walking in rural areas. *American Journal of Preventive Medicine, 27* (1), 28-34.

Brownson, R.C., Baker, E.A., Housemann, R.A., Brennan, L.K., & Bacak, S.J. (2001). Environmental and policy determinants of physical activity in the United States. *American Journal of Public Health, 91* (12), 1995-2003.

Brownson, R.C., Hoehner, C.M., Brennan, L.K., Cook, R.A., Elliott, M.B., & McMullen, K.M. (2004). Reliability of two instruments for auditing the environment for physical activity. *Journal of Physical Activity and Health, 1,* 189-207.

Centers for Disease Control and Prevention. (2007). StairWELL to Better Health. Retrieved May 29, 2007, from www.cdc.gov/nccdphp/dnpa/hwi/toolkits/stairwell/index.htm

Craig, C.L., Brownson, R.C., Cragg, S.E., & Dunn, A.L. (2002). Exploring the effect of the environment on physical activity: A study examining walking to work. *American Journal of Preventive Medicine, 23* (2S), 36-43.

Cunningham, G.O., & Michael Y.L. (2004). Concepts guiding the study of the impact of the built environment on physical activity for older adults: A review of the literature. *American Journal of Health Promotion, 18* (6), 435-443.

Evenson, K.R., Herring, A.H., & Huston, S.L. (2005). Evaluating change in physical activity with the building of a multi-use trail. *American Journal of Preventive Medicine, 28* (2), 177-185.

Ewing, R., Schmid, T., Killingsworth, R., Zlot, A., & Raudenbush, S. (2003). Relationship between urban sprawl and physical activity, obesity, and morbidity. *American Journal of Health Promotion, 18* (1), 47-57.

Giles-Corti, B., Broomhall, M.H., Knuiman, M., Collins, C., Douglas, K., Ng, K., Lange, A., & Donovan, R.J. (2005). How important is distance to, attractiveness, and size of public open space? *American Journal of Preventive Medicine, 28* (2S), 169-176.

Gordon-Larsen, P., Nelson, M.C., Page, P., & Popkin, B.M. (2006). Inequality in the built environment underlies key health disparities in physical activity and obesity. *Pediatrics, 117* (2), 417-424.

Handy, S., Cao, X., & Mokhtarian, P.L. (2006). Self-selection in the relationship between the built environment and walking: Evidence from Northern California. *Journal of the American Planning Association, 72* (1), 55-74.

Huston, S.L., Evenson, K.R., Bors, P., & Gizlice, Z. (2003). Neighborhood environment, access to places for activity, and leisure-time physical activity in a diverse North Carolina population. *American Journal of Health Promotion, 18* (1), 58-69.

Moudon, A.V., & Drewnowski, A. (2005). Fat neighborhoods: Spatial epidemiology meets urban form. Retrieved May 29, 2007, from www.nwephp.org/nph

National Center for Health Statistics. (1994). NHC plan and operation of the Third National Health and Nutrition Examination Survey, 1988-1994. *Vital Health Statistics, 1* (32).

Parks, S.E., Housemann, R.A., & Brownson, R.C. (2003). Differential correlates of physical activity in urban and rural adults of various socioeconomic backgrounds in the United States. *Journal of Epidemiology in Community Health, 57,* 29-35.

Porter, D.E., Kirtland, K.A., Neet, M.J., Williams, J.E., & Ainsworth, B.E. (2004). Considerations for using a Geographic Information System to assess environmental supports for physical activity. Preventing chronic disease. Retrieved October 2004 from www.cdc.gov/pcd/issues/2004

Robert Wood Johnson Foundation. (2007). The Synthesis Project: New insights from research results. The built environment and physical activity: What is the relationship? Retrieved April 12, 2007, from www.policysynthesis.org

Saelens, B.E., Sallis, J.F., Black, J.B., & Chen, D. (2003). Neighborhood-based differences in physical activity: An environment scale evaluation. *American Journal of Public Health, 93* (9), 1552-1558.

Sallis, J.F., & Owen, N. (1997). Ecological models. In K. Glanz, F.M. Lewis, & B.K. Rimer (Eds.), *Health behavior and health education* (pp. 403-424). San Francisco, CA: Jossey-Bass.

Sharpe, P.A., Granner, M.L., Hutto, B., & Ainsworth, B.E. (2004). Association of environmental factors to meeting physical activity recommendations in two South Carolina counties. *American Journal of Health Promotion, 18* (3), 251-257.

Troped, P.J., Saunders, R.P., Pate, R.R., Reininger, B., & Addy, C.L. (2003). Correlates of recreational and transportation physical activity among adults in a New England community. *Preventive Medicine, 37* (4), 304-310.

U.S. Department of Health and Human Services. (2000). *Healthy People 2010: Understanding and improving health.* Washington, DC: U.S. Government Printing Office.

Webb, O.J., & Eves, F.F. (2007). Promoting stair climbing: Effects of message specificity and validation. *Health Education Research, 22* (1), 49-57.

Wilcox, S., Castro, C., King, A.C., Housemann, R., & Brownson, R.C. (2000). Determinants of leisure time physical activity in rural compared with urban older and ethnically diverse women in the United States. *Journal of Epidemiology in Community Health, 54,* 667-672.

Young, D.R., & Voorhees, C.C. (2003). Personal, social, and physical environmental correlates of physical activity in urban African-American women. *American Journal of Preventive Medicine, 25* (3), 38-44.

Chapter 9

Aarnio, M., Winter, T., Kujala, U.M., & Kaprio, J. (1997). Familial aggregation of leisure-time physical activity—A three generation study. *International Journal of Sports Medicine, 18,* 549-556.

Addley, K., McQuillan, P., & Ruddle, M. (2001). Creating healthy workplaces in Northern Ireland: Evaluation of a lifestyle and physical activity assessment programme. *Occupational Medicine, 51* (7), 439-449.

Aittasalo, M., Miilunpalo, S., Stahl, T., & Kukkonen-Harjula, K. (2006). From innovation to practice: Initiation, implementation, and evaluation of a physician-based physical activity promotion program in Finland. *Health Promotion International, 22* (1), 19-27.

Amani-Golshani, N. (2006). Exercise as medicine. *Fitness Business Canada, 7* (6), 34-36.

Bagley, S., Salmon, J., & Crawford, D. (2006). Family structure and children's television viewing and physical activity. *Medicine & Science in Sports & Exercise, 38* (5), 910-918.

Bar-Or, O., Foreyt, J., Bouchard, C., Brownell, K.D., Dietz, W.H., Ravussin, E., Salbe, A.D., Schwenger, S., St Jeor, S., & Torun, B. (1998). Physical activity, genetic and nutritional considerations in childhood weight management. *Medicine & Science in Sports & Exercise, 30,* 2-10.

Beunen, G., & Thomis, M. (1999). Genetic determinants of sports participation and daily physical activity. *International Journal of Obesity, 23* (Suppl. 3), S55-S63.

Bonomi, A.E., Boudreau, D.M., Fishman, P.A., Meenan, R.T., & Revicki, D.A. (2005). Is a family equal to the sum of its parts? Estimating family-level well-being for cost effectiveness analysis. *Quality of Life Research, 14* (4), 1127-1133.

Bopp, M., Wilcox, S., Laken, M., Hooker, S.P., Saunders, R., Parra-Medina, D., Butler, K., & McClorin, L. (2007). Using the RE-AIM framework to evaluate a physical activity intervention in churches. *Preventing Chronic Disease, 4* (4). Retrieved October 26, 2007, from www.cdc.gov/pcd/issues/2007/oct/06_0155.htm

Bull, F.C.L., Schipper, E.C.C., Jamrozik, K., & Blanksby, B.A. (1997). How can and do Australian doctors promote physical activity? *Preventive Medicine, 26,* 866-873.

Carmeli, E., Sheklow, S.L., & Coleman, R. (2006). A comparative study of organized class-based exercise programs versus individual home-based exercise programs for elderly patients following hip surgery. *Disability and Rehabilitation, 28* (16), 997-1005.

Clocksin, B.D., Watson, D.L., & Ransdell, L. (2002). Understanding youth obesity and media use: Implications for future intervention programs. *Quest, 54* (4), 259-275.

Dishman, R.K., Oldenburg, B., O'Neal, H., & Shephard, R.J. (1998). Worksite physical activity interventions. *American Journal of Preventive Medicine, 15* (4), 344-361.

Douglas, F., Torrance, N., van Teijlingen, E., Meloni, S., & Kerr, A. (2006). Primary care staff's views and experiences related to routinely advising patients about physical activity. A questionnaire survey. *BMC Public Health, 6*: 138. Retrieved October 28, 2007, from www.biomedcentral.com/1471-2458-6-138

Eakin, E.C., Brown, W.J., Marshall, A.L., Mummery, K., & Larsen, E. (2004). Physical activity promotion in primary care: Bridging the gap between research and practice. *American Journal of Preventive Medicine, 27* (4), 297-303.

Elley, C.R., Kerse, N., Arroll, B., & Robinson, E. (2003). Effectiveness of counseling patients on physical activity in general practice: Cluster randomized controlled trial. *British Medical Journal, 326*, 793. Retrieved October 28, 2007, from www.bmj.com/cgi/reprint/326/7393/793

Fitzgibbon, M.L., Stolley, M.R., Ganschow, P., Schiffer, L., Wells, A., Simon, N., & Dyer, A. (2005). Results of a faith-based weight loss intervention for Black women. *Journal of the National Medical Association, 97* (10), 1393-1402.

Flora, P.K., & Faulkner, G.E.J. (2006). Physical activity: An innovative context for intergenerational programming. *Journal of Intergenerational Relationships, 4* (4), 63-74.

Fogelholm, M., Nuutinen, O., Pasanen, M., Myohanen, E., & Saatela, T. (1999). Parent-child relationship of physical activity patterns and obesity. *International Journal of Obesity and Related Metabolic Disorders, 23* (12), 1262-1268.

Harden, A., Peersman, G., Oliver, S., Mauthen, M., & Oakley, A. (1999). A systematic review of the effectiveness of health promotion interventions in the workplace. *Occupational Medicine, 49* (8), 540-548. Retrieved November 10, 2007, from http://occmed.oxfordjournals.org/cgi/reprint/49/8/540

Hatch, J., Cunningham, A., Woods, W., & Snipes, F. (1986). The Fitness Through Churches project: Description of a community-based cardiovascular health promotion intervention. *Hygie, 5* (3), 9-12.

Higgins, M. (2000). Epidemiology and prevention of coronary heart disease in families. *American Journal of Medicine, 108*, 387-395.

Hopper, C.A., Munoz, K.D., Gruber, M.B., & Nguyen, K.P. (2005). The effects of a family fitness program on the physical activity and nutrition behaviors of third-grade children. *Research Quarterly for Exercise and Sport, 76* (2), 130-140.

Keays, S.L., Bullock-Saxton, J.E., Newcombe, P., & Bullock, M.I. (2006). The effectiveness of a preoperative home-based physiotherapy programme for chronic anterior cruciate ligament deficiency. *Physiotherapy Research International, 11* (4), 204-218.

Knutsen, S.F., & Knutsen, R. (1991). The Tromso Survey: The Family Intervention Study. The effect of intervention on some coronary risk factors and dietary habits: A 6-year follow-up. *Preventive Medicine, 20*, 197-212.

Lasater, T.M., Wells, B.L., Carleton, R.A., & Elder, J.P. (1986). The role of churches in disease prevention research studies. *Public Health Reports, 101* (2), 125-131.

Leaf, D.A., & Reuben, D.B. (1996). Lifestyle interventions for promoting physical activity: A kilocalorie expenditure-based home feasibility study. *American Journal of the Medical Sciences, 312* (2), 68-75.

Mayoux-Benhamou, M.A., Roux, C., Perraud, A., Fermanian, J., Rahali-Kachlouf, H., & Revel, M. (2005). Predictors of compliance with a home-based exercise program added to usual medical care in preventing postmenopausal osteoporosis: An 18 month prospective study. *Osteoporosis International, 16* (3), 325-331.

Peterson, J., Atwood, J.R., & Yates, B. (2002). Key elements for church-based health promotion programs: Outcome-based literature review. *Public Health Nursing, 19* (6), 401-411.

Petrella, R.J., & Bartha, C. (2000). Home based exercise therapy for older patients with knee osteoarthritis: A randomized clinical trial. *Journal of Rheumatology, 27*, 2215-2221.

Pinto, B.M., Frierson, G.M., Rabin, C., Trunzo, J.J., & Marcus, B.H. (2005). Home-based physical activity intervention for breast cancer patients. *Journal of Clinical Oncology, 23* (15), 3577-3587.

Plotnikoff, R.C., Brunet, S., Courneya, K.S., Spence, J.C., Birkett, N.J., Marcus, B., & Whiteley, J. (2007). The efficacy of stage-matched and standard public health materials for promoting physical activity in the workplace: The Physical Activity Workplace Study (PAWS). *American Journal of Health Promotion, 21* (6), 501-509.

Pollner, M., & Stein, J. (1996). Narrative mapping of social worlds: The voice of experience in alcoholics anonymous. *Symbolic Interaction, 19*, 203-223.

Pyke, S.D., Wood, D.A., Kinmonth, A.L., & Thompson, S.G. (1997). Change in coronary risk and coronary risk factor levels in couples following lifestyle intervention. The British Family Heart Study. *Archives of Family Medicine, 6*, 354-360.

Ransdell, L.B., & Rehling, S.L. (1996). Church-based health promotion: A review of the current literature. *American Journal of Health Behavior, 20* (4), 195-207.

Ransdell, L.B., Robertson, L., Ornes, L., & Moyer-Mileur, L. (2004). Generations exercising together to improve fitness (GET FIT): A pilot study designed to increase physical activity and improve health-related fitness in three generations of women. *Women & Health, 40* (3), 77-94.

Redmond, C., Spoth, R., Shin, C., & Lepper, H.S. (1999). Modeling long-term parent outcomes of two universal family-focused preventive interventions: One-year follow-up results. *Journal of Consulting and Clinical Psychology, 67* (6), 975-984.

Ribera, A.P., McKenna, J., & Riddoch, C. (2006). Physical activity promotion in general practices of Barcelona: A case study. *Health Education Research, 21* (4), 538-548.

Ritchie, L.D., Welk, G., Styne, D., Gerstein, D.E., Crawford, P.B. (2005). Family environment and pediatric overweight: What is a parent to do? *Journal of the American Dietetic Association, 105* (5 Suppl. 1), S70-S79.

Robertson, M.C., Devlin, N., Gardner, M.M., & Campbell, A.J. (2001). Effectiveness and economic evaluation of a nurse delivered home exercise programme to prevent falls: Randomised controlled trial. *British Medical Journal, 322* (24), 1-6.

Rodearmel, S.J., Wyatt, H.R., Barry, M.J., Dong, F., Pan, D., Israel, R.G., Cho, S.S., McBurney, M.I., & Hill, J.O. (2006). A family-based approach to preventing excessive weight gain. *Obesity, 14* (8), 1392-1401.

Rodearmel, S.J., Wyatt, H.R., Stroebele, N., Smith, S.M., Ogden, L.G., & Hill, J.O. (2007). Small changes in dietary sugar and physical activity as an approach to preventing excessive weight gain: The America on the Move Family Study. *Pediatrics, 120* (4), e869-e879.

Rohm-Young, D., & Stewart, K.J. (2006). A church-based physical activity intervention for African American women. *Family & Community Health, 29* (2), 103-117.

Rose, S.B., Lawton, B.A., Elley, C.R., Dowell, A.C., & Fenton A.J. (2007). The Women's Lifestyle Study, 2-year randomized controlled trial of physical activity counseling in primary health care: Rationale and study design. *BMC Public Health, 7*, 166. Retrieved October 28, 2007, from www.biomedcentral.com/content/pdf/1471-2458-7-166.pdf

Salmon, J., Timperio, A., Telford, A., Carver, A., & Crawford, D. (2005). Association of family environment with children's television viewing and with low level of physical activity. *Obesity Research, 13* (11), 1939-1951.

Taggart, A.C., Taggart, J., & Siedentop, D. (1986). Effects of a home-based activity program: A study with low fitness elementary school children. *Behavior Modification, 10* (4), 487-507.

Taylor, A. (2003). The role of primary care in promoting physical activity. In J. McKenna, C. Riddoch, & P. Bassingstoke (Eds.), *Perspectives on health and exercise* (pp. 153-173). New York: Macmillan.

Tessaro, I.A., Taylor, S., Belton, L., Campbell, M.K., Benedict, S., Kelsey, K., & DeVellis, B. (2000). Adapting a natural (lay) helpers model of change for worksite health promotion for women. *Health Education Research, 15* (5), 603-614.

Teufel-Shone, N.I., Drummond, R., & Rawiel, U. (2005). Developing and adapting a family-based diabetes program at the U.S.-Mexico border. *Preventing Chronic Disease: Public Health Research, Practice, and Policy* (serial online), *2* (1), 1-9. Retrieved July 6, 2007, from www.cdc.gov/pcd/issues/2005/jan/04_0083.htm

Thomas, L., & Williams, M. (2006). Promoting physical activity in the workplace: Using pedometers to increase daily activity levels. *Health Promotion Journal of Australia, 17* (2), 97-102.

Tuzin, B.J., Mulvihill, M.M., Kilbourn, K.M., Bertran, D.A., Buono, M., Hovell, M.F., Harwood, I.R., & Light, M.L. (1998). Increasing physical activity of children with cystic fibrosis: A home-based family intervention. *Pediatric Exercise Science, 10*, 57-68.

Wells, B.L., DePue, J.D., Lasater, T.M., & Carleton, R.A. (1988). A report on church site weight control. *Health Education Research, 3* (3), 305-316.

Wilbur, J., Miller, A.M., Chandler, P., & McDevitt, J. (2003). Determinants of physical activity and adherence to a 24-week home-based walking program in African American and Caucasian women. *Research in Nursing and Health, 26,* 213-224.

Wilcox, S., Laken, M., Anderson, T., Bopp, M., Bryant, D., Carter, R., Gethers, O., Jordan, J., McClorin, L., O'Rourke, K., Parrott, A.W., Swinton, R., & Yancey, A. (2007). The Health-e-AME faith-based physical activity initiative: Description and baseline findings. *Health Promotion Practice, 8* (1), 69-78.

Wrotniak, B.H., Epstein, L.H., Paluch, R.A., & Roemmich, J.N. (2005). Parent weight change as a predictor of child weight change in family-based behavioral obesity treatment. *Archives of Pediatric and Adolescent Medicine, 158,* 342-347.

Wynne, R., & Clarkin, N. (1992). *Under construction—Building for health in the EC workplace.* Luxembourg: European Foundation for the Improvement of Living and Working Conditions.

Zion, A.S., De Meersman, R., Diamond, B.E., & Bloomfield, D.M. (2003). A home-based resistance training program using elastic bands for elderly patients with orthostatic hypotension. *Clinical Autonomic Research, 13,* 286-292.

Chapter 10

Bauman, A.E, Bellew, B., Owen, N., & Vita, P. (2001). Impact of an Australian mass media campaign targeting physical activity in 1998. *American Journal of Preventive Medicine, 21* (1), 41-47.

Brown, W.J., Eakin, E., Mummery, K., & Trost, S.G. (2003). 10,000 Steps Rockhampton: Establishing a multi-strategy physical activity promotion project in a community. *Health Promotion Journal of Australia, 14* (2), 95-100.

Bull, F.C., Kreuter, M.W., & Scharff, D.P. (1999). Effects of tailored, personalized and general health messages on physical activity. *Patient Education and Counseling, 36,* 181-192.

Cameron, R., Bauman, A., & Rose, A. (2006). Innovations in population intervention research capacity: The contributions of Canada on the Move. *Canadian Journal of Public Health, 97* (Suppl. 1), S5-S9.

Cavill, N., & Bauman, A. (2004). Changing the way people think about health-enhancing physical activity: Do mass media campaigns have a role? *Journal of Sport Sciences, 22,* 771-790.

Craig, C.L., Cragg, S.E., Tudor-Locke, C., & Bauman, A. (2006). Proximal impact of Canada on the Move: The relationship of campaign awareness to pedometer ownership and use. *Canadian Journal of Public Health, 97* (Suppl. 1), S21-S27.

Demark-Wahnefried, W., Clipp, E.C., Lipkus, I.M., Lobach, D., Clutter-Snyder, D., Sloane, R., Peterson, B., Macri, J.M., Rock, C.L., McBride, C.M., & Kraus, W.E. (2007). Main outcomes of the FRESH START trial: A sequentially tailored, diet and exercise mailed print intervention among breast and prostate cancer survivors. *Journal of Clinical Oncology, 25* (19), 2709-2718.

Dietz, W.H. (2006). Canada on the Move: A novel effort to increase physical activity among Canadians. *Canadian Journal of Public Health, 97* (Suppl. 1), S3-S4.

Dishman, R.K., & Buckworth, J. (1996). Increasing physical activity: A quantitative synthesis. *Medicine & Science in Sports & Exercise, 28,* 706-719.

Eads, S. (2007 Autumn/Winter). Podcasts: Your portable trainer. *Body Sense,* 36-37.

Eakin, E.G., Brown, W.J., Marshall, A.L., Mummery, K., & Larsen, E. (2004). Physical activity promotion in primary care: Bridging the gap between research and practice. *American Journal of Preventive Medicine, 27* (4), 297-303.

Eakin, E.G., Mummery, K., Reeves, M.M., Lawler, S.P., Schofield, G., Marshall, A.J., & Brown, W.J. (2007). Correlates of pedometer use: Results from a community-based physical activity intervention trial (10,000 Steps Rockhampton). *International Journal of Behavioral Nutrition and Physical Activity, 4,* 31.

Faulkner, G., & Finlay, S.J. (2006). Canada on the Move: An intensive media analysis from inception to reception. *Canadian Journal of Public Health, 97* (Suppl. 1), S16-S20.

Ferney, S.L., & Marshall, A.L. (2006). Website physical activity interventions: Preferences of potential users. *Health Education Research, 21* (4), 560-566.

Fogg, B.J. (2003). *Persuasive technology: Using computers to change what we think and do.* San Francisco, CA: Morgan Kaufmann.

Hartman, J.M., & Jackson, B.H. (2007 January). Podcasting. *IDEA Fitness Journal,* 30-32.

Huhman, M.E., Potter, L.D., Duke, J.C., Judkins, D.R., Heitzler, C.D., & Wong, F.L. (2007). Evaluation of a national physical activity intervention for children: VERB™ Campaign, 2002-2004. *American Journal of Preventive Medicine, 32* (1), 38-43.

Hurling, R., Catt, M., DeBoni, M., Fairley, B.W., Hurst, T., Murray, P., Richardson, A., & Singh-Sodhi, J. (2007). Using internet and mobile phone technology to deliver an automated physical activity program: Randomized controlled trial. *Journal of Medical Internet Research, 9* (2), e7.

Hurling, R., Fairley, B.W., & Dias, M.B. (2006). Internet-based exercise intervention systems: Are more interactive designs better? *Psychology and Health, 21* (6), 757-772.

Lombard, D.N., Lombard, T., & Winett, R.A. (1995). Walking to meet health guidelines: The effect of prompting frequency and prompt structure. *Health Psychology, 14,* 164-170.

Mailbach, E. (2007). The influence of the media environment on physical activity: Looking for the big picture. *American Journal of Health Promotion, 21* (4 Suppl.), 353-362.

Marcus, B.H., Lewis, B.A., Williams, D.M., Dunsiger, S., Jakicic, J.M., Whiteley, J.A., Albrecht, A.E., Napolitano, M.A., Bock, B.C., Tate, D.F., Sciamanna, C.N., & Parisi, A.F. (2007). A comparison of internet and print-based physical activity interventions. *Archives of Internal Medicine, 167,* 944-949.

Marcus, B.H., Napolitano, M.A., Lewis, B.A., Whiteley, J.A., Albrecht, A., Parisi, A., Bock, B., Pinto, B., Sciamanna, C., King, A.C., Jakicic, J., & Papandonatos, G.D. (2007). Telephone versus print delivery of an individualized motivationally tailored physical activity intervention: Project STRIDE. *Health Psychology, 26* (4), 401-409.

Marcus, B.H., Owen, N., Forsyth, L., Cavill, N.A., & Fridinger, F. (1998). Physical activity interventions using mass media, print media, and information technology. *American Journal of Preventive Medicine, 15* (4), 362-378.

Marks, J.T., Campbell, M.K., Ward, D.S., Ribisl, K.M., Wildemuth, B.M., & Symons, M.J. (2006). A comparison of web and print media for physical activity promotion among adolescent girls. *Journal of Adolescent Health, 39* (1), 96-104.

Marshall, A.L., Eakin, E.G, Leslie, E.R., & Owen, N. (2005). Exploring the feasibility of using internet technology to promote physical activity within a defined community. *Health Promotion Journal of Australia, 16* (1), 82-84.

Marshall, A.L., Leslie, E.R., Bauman, A.E., Marcus, B.H., & Owen, N. (2003). Print versus website physical activity programs: A randomized trial. *American Journal of Preventive Medicine, 25* (2), 88-94.

Marshall, A.L., Owen, N., & Bauman, A.E. (2004). Mediated approaches for influencing physical activity: Update of the evidence on mass media, print, telephone, and website delivery of interventions. *Journal of Science and Medicine in Sport, 7* (1 Suppl.), 74-80.

Mummery, W.K., Schofield, G., Hinchliffe, A., Joyner, K., & Brown, W. (2006). Dissemination of a community-based physical activity project: The case of 10,000 steps. *Journal of Science and Medicine in Sport, 9* (5), 424-430.

Napolitano, M.A., & Marcus, B.H. (2002). Targeting and tailoring physical activity information using print and information technologies. *Exercise and Sport Science Reviews, 30* (3), 122-128.

Peterson, M., Abraham, A., & Waterfield, A. (2005). Marketing physical activity: Lessons learned from a statewide media campaign. *Health Promotion Practice, 6* (4), 437-446.

Ransdell, L.B., Taylor, A., Oakland, D., Schmidt, J., Moyer-Mileur, L., & Shultz, B. (2003). Daughters and mothers exercising together: Effects of home- and community based programs. *Medicine & Science in Sports & Exercise, 35* (2), 286-296.

Reger, B., Cooper, L., Booth-Butterfield, S., Smith, H., Bauman, A., Wootan, M., Middlestadt, S., Marcus, B., & Greer, F. (2002). Wheeling Walks: A community campaign using paid media to encourage walking among sedentary adults. *Preventive Medicine, 35,* 285-292.

Rovniak, L.S., Hovell, M.F., Wojcik, J.R., Winett, R.A., Martinez-Donate, A.P. (2005). Enhancing theoretical fidelity: An e-mail-based walking program demonstration. *American Journal of Health Promotion, 20* (2), 85-95.

Schultz, S.J. (1993). Educational and behavioral strategies related to knowledge of and participation in an exercise program after cardiac positron emission tomography. *Patient Education and Counseling, 22,* 47-57.

Sevick, M.A., Napolitano, M.A., Papandonatos, G.D., Gordon, A.J., Reiser, L.M., & Marcus, B.H. (2007). Cost-effectiveness of alternative approaches for motivating activity in sedentary adults: Results of Project STRIDE. *Preventive Medicine, 45,* 54-61.

Tate, D.F., Wing, R.R., & Winett, R.A. (2001). Using internet technology to deliver a behavioral weight loss program. *Journal of the American Medical Association, 289,* 1172-1177.

Wantland, D.J., Portillo, C.J., Holzemer, W.L., Slaughter, R., & McGhee, E.M. (2004). The effectiveness of web-based vs. non-web-based interventions: A meta-analysis of behavioral change outcomes. *Journal of Medical Internet Research, 6* (4), e40.

INDEX

Note: The italicized *f* and *t* following page numbers refer to figures and tables, respectively.

A

accelerometers 29–30
Active Living intervention 160–161
Active Living Resources Center 111–112
addictive foods 63
adherence rates, home-based programs 117
aerobics 88
  church-based programs 131–132
aesthetics, stairwell interventions 104
African Americans. *See* ethnic populations
African American Women Fight Cancer With Fitness (FCF) 47
AHA/ACSM Health/Fitness Facility Preparticipation Screening Questionnaire 68
Alaska Native 92–93
all-cause mortality scientific studies 8–9
American College of Sports Medicine 4–5, 7
American Diabetes Association 63
American Heart Association 7
American Indians 92–93
America on the Move 161
appearance, stairwell interventions 104
Asian Americans 93–94
assessment, data collection 14–16
attractiveness, neighborhood 106

B

barriers to physical activity. *see also* decisional balance
  church-based physical activity programs 130–131

family-based programs 125–126
home-based physical activity programs 117–118
mediated interventions 155–157
medical community-based physical activity programs 135–136
overcoming strategies 61, 62*t*
overweight and obesity interventions 61, 62*t*
women interventions 40–43, 41*t*–42*t*
worksite-based physical activity programs 139–140
behavior modification, worksite-based programs 139
body fat 50
  percentage 50–51
body mass index (BMI) 50–51
Buckworth, J. xv
built environment 102, 102*t*

C

caloric expenditures 57*t*
Canada on the Move 161
Canadian Institutes of Health Research 161
cancer scientific studies 9–10
cardiovascular disease (CVD) scientific studies 9
Cardiovascular Health and Activity Maintenance Program (CHAMP) 79
chair exercises 133
children, overweight 51
church-based physical activity programs 129–131
  aerobic fitness program 131–132

ABOUT THE AUTHORS

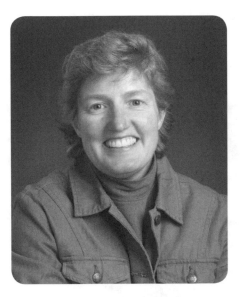

Lynda B. Ransdell, PhD, is a professor in the department of kinesiology at Boise State University.

Ransdell has dedicated her career and research to helping sedentary people increase their levels of physical activity. Ransdell has designed, implemented, and evaluated numerous physical activity interventions and has worked as a consultant to help others develop interventions in community settings.

Known for her research of physical activity patterns of women, Ransdell has conducted two well-respected studies, Daughters and Mothers Exercising Together (DAMET) and Generations Exercising Together to Improve Fitness (GET FIT), which detail some of the only family-based interventions known to be successful in increasing physical activity in typically inactive women.

Ransdell has published over 60 peer-reviewed articles and 14 book chapters, mostly related to increasing physical activity in sedentary individuals. She is also the author of *Ensuring the Health of Active and Athletic Girls and Women*, a popular text for courses examining the physiological and psychological implications of sport and physical activity participation for girls and women.

She is a fellow of the American College of Sports Medicine (ACSM) and the Research Consortium of the American Alliance for Health, Physical Education, Recreation and Dance. Ransdell has also served as president of the National Association for Girls and Women in Sport, editor of the *Women in Sport and Physical Activity Journal,* and coeditor of *Physical Activity Today*. She is the recipient of the ACSM Visiting Scholar award from University of South Carolina (1998) and Outstanding Alumni awards from Arizona State University and Eastern Kentucky University.

Ransdell resides in Boise, Idaho, where she enjoys participating in ice hockey, cross-country skiing, running, and mountain biking.

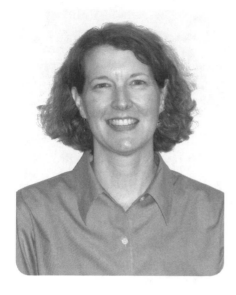

Mary K. Dinger, PhD, is a professor in the department of health and exercise science at the University of Oklahoma at Norman, where her teaching and research focus on promoting physical activity.

Working in a research, consulting, or community service capacity, Dinger has designed, implemented, and evaluated several physical activity interventions. She has published her research in more than 50 articles in peer-reviewed journals.

Dinger is a fellow of both the American College of Sports Medicine (ACSM) and the Research Consortium of the American Alliance for Health, Physical Education, Recreation and Dance (AAHPERD). She currently serves as epidemiology section editor for *Research Quarterly for Exercise and Sport* and on the editorial board of the *American Journal of Health Behavior*. She was previously an editorial board member of the *American Journal of Health Education* and an executive board member of the American Academy of Health Behavior and the Research Consortium of AAHPERD.

Dinger resides in Norman, Oklahoma. She enjoys staying physically active by playing with her daughter, biking, and hiking.

Jennifer Huberty, PhD, is an assistant professor in the department of health, physical education, and recreation at the University of Nebraska at Omaha, where she manages the graduate curriculum for physical activity in health promotion.

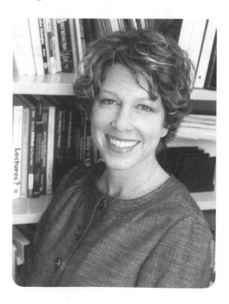

Huberty has designed, implemented, and evaluated numerous research- and community-based physical activity interventions. She is the creator of Women Bound to Be Active, a physical activity book club aimed at increasing the number of women who maintain healthy physical activity behaviors. This nine-month intervention provides women with the skills and tools for initiating and maintaining a physically active lifestyle. The rationale for this program and details on its feasibility have been published in *Research Quarterly* and *Women and Health*.

Based on research gathered in Women Bound to Be Active, Huberty also created a locally implemented weight management program, Fit for Life, which provides a no-cost opportunity for underserved people to learn healthy behaviors and be active within their communities. Huberty directs the physical activity component for Club Possible, a physical activity and nutrition education afterschool program focusing on prevention of childhood obesity. The program has been implemented in 18 afterschool agencies, including CampFire USA, YMCA, Boys and Girls Club, and Girl Scouts.

Huberty is a member of the Society of Behavioral Medicine and the American Alliance for Health, Physical Education, Recreation and Dance. For outstanding research and community service, Huberty was awarded the Varner Professorship for 2007. In 1999, she received a graduate student research award from the Southern Academy for Women in Physical Activity, Sport, and Health.

Huberty resides in LaVista, Nebraska, with her husband, Rodger. She enjoys Spinning, running, weight training, and scrapbooking in her free time.

Kim H. Miller, PhD, is an associate professor of health promotion in the department of kinesiology and health promotion at the University of Kentucky at Lexington, where she works with undergraduate and graduate students to design and implement health promotion interventions.

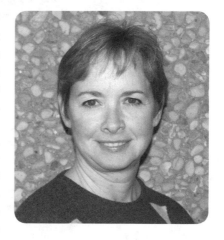

Miller received her doctorate in health education from Southern Illinois University in 2000. For over eight years, she has conducted research in the area of health and physical activity, publishing numerous research papers and presenting her findings at international conferences. Miller has also served as a consultant in designing physical activity and health promotion interventions for employee wellness programs in a variety of settings. She is a member of the American Academy of Health Behavior and the American Association for Health Education.

In her free time, she enjoys running, hiking, reading, and cooking. Miller resides in Lexington, Kentucky.

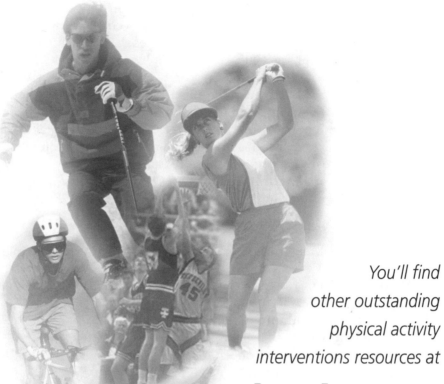

*You'll find
other outstanding
physical activity
interventions resources at*

www.HumanKinetics.com

In the U.S. call

1-800-747-4457

Australia..............................08 8372 0999
Canada..............................1-800-465-7301
Europe......................+44 (0) 113 255 5665
New Zealand...................0064 9 448 1207

HUMAN KINETICS
The Information Leader in Physical Activity
P.O. Box 5076 • Champaign, IL 61825-5076 USA